BOTOX®

BOTOX®

*Everything You Need to Know About the Amazing
New Anti-Wrinkle Treatment*

RON M. SHELTON, M.D.,
AND
TERRY MALLOY

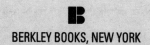

BERKLEY BOOKS, NEW YORK

BOTOX®

A Berkley Book / published by arrangement with
the author

Botox is a registered trademark of Allergan, Inc.

This book is not authorized, approved, licensed
or endorsed by Allergan, Inc.

PRINTING HISTORY
Berkley edition / October 2002

Visit our website at
www.penguinputnam.com

ISBN: 0-425-18917-1

BERKLEY®
Berkley Books are published by The Berkley Publishing Group,
a division of Penguin Putnam Inc.,
375 Hudson Street, New York, New York 10014.
BERKLEY and the "B" design
are trademarks belonging to Penguin Putnam Inc.

PRINTED IN THE UNITED STATES OF AMERICA

10 9 8 7 6 5 4 3

Contents

Acknowledgments

The authors would like to acknowledge the highly supportive assistance and guidance of our agent, Madeline Morel, and our editor, Christine Zika. Sincere and heartfelt thanks to both!

Introduction

It's been called "the coffee-break face-lift," "the miracle drug for boomers," "the New Age Fountain of Youth," and "the most popular cosmetic medical procedure in the country." You've heard about it, read about it, watched talk shows about it, and been amazed by the suddenly youthful appearances of countless celebrities who use it.

Perhaps you have friends who've tried it and you can't get over the fantastic results. Millions of people—women and men—seem to swear by it.

But is Botox really the magic potion that so many seem to think? How can it be safe if it is made from the same toxin that can cause the potentially fatal disease botulism?

You know that Botox wears off and the procedure has to be repeated if you want the rejuvenating effects to last. Is there any evidence that repeated use over years can build up the toxin in your body and eventually cause health problems?

Can Botox treat all the cosmetic problems on your face that make you look so much older? Frown lines, crow's-feet, smile folds, forehead lines, chin depressions? Or only some of them?

Can anyone give you Botox? Your dentist? Your beautician? Or is it best to see only a specially trained dermatologist, plastic surgeon, or ophthalmologist?

Are the increasingly popular "Botox parties" a good idea? Could you have problems if you have a few drinks and then get a Botox treatment at your friend's house or in a beauty salon?

With all the media hype over Botox, almost everyone has heard about it by now. So it's natural to assume you know everything you need to know, and if you have some facial lines or wrinkles you want to eliminate, it seems simple enough to spend ten minutes of your time banishing them with a few little injections.

But it really isn't that simple.

Botox is a drug, and Botox injections are serious medical procedures. True, they are not major surgery, but as with any medical treatment, the better informed you are, the better your results will be.

And there's a great deal to learn about Botox. In this book you will discover:

- How Botox was developed

- The medical uses for Botox

- The cosmetic uses for Botox

- How to determine if you are a good candidate

- Who should not use Botox

- How to find the best doctor

- What happens, step-by-step, in the doctor's office

- What kinds of results you can expect

- What precautions you must take following treatment

- The possible side effects and dangers, including pain

- What to do if you don't get the results you want or if you don't get any results at all

- When to go back for further treatments

- The cost of treatment and whether insurance covers it

- What other cosmetic medical treatments are available for facial rejuvenation, and which ones can be used in conjunction with Botox for maximum effect

- What other drugs are on the horizon

- A dermatologist's program for lifelong skin care

- Where to go for further information

So whether you have never had a Botox treatment and are now thinking about it, have already had one or more treatments and want to know more about it, know someone who is trying to decide whether to try it, or are just plain curious to learn more about this groundbreaking facial transformer, this book will provide you with much-needed information about Botox, the "billion-dollar drug."

Written by a cosmetic dermatologist with close to ten years of extensive experience with Botox, and a seasoned health and medical writer, this book will be your guide to everything you want to know about Botox. It will help you decide whether it's safe, whether it can help your specific skin problems, and whether you want to explore it further and possibly try it, or continue with your present treatments.

Celebrities and the jet set have been using Botox for many years. Only now, with the recent FDA (U.S. Government Food and Drug Administration) approval for cosmetic use, has widespread publicity made this amazing drug known and available to the average person.

Today, secretaries, librarians, account executives, teachers, firemen, homemakers, contractors, salespeople, and everyone else can enjoy a relatively inexpensive, nonsurgical brow-lift. They can walk in, undergo a brief session in the doctor's office, and quickly begin to look years younger.

Botox is not for everyone and does not work for every sign of aging on your face. But if you are a good candidate and if you want to invest in this procedure, the chances are excellent that you, like so many other millions of people, will be thrilled with the results.

This book, written in easily accessible question-and-answer format, is like a pleasant and informative visit with your doctor. Using his long-term experience with Botox and with hundreds of Botox patients, Dr. Ron Shelton provides complete, essential, and easy-to-understand information to help you learn about every aspect of Botox and determine if it's right for you.

So come along with us and learn more about Botox, "the super smoother" that can change your life.

Chapter 1

Why Does Your Skin Age?

Before we can understand how Botox works (or does not work), we need to know a little about our skin.

In this chapter, we will find out what composes the skin, why signs of aging begin to appear, and why some people show more signs of aging than others. We will also learn which factors, other than the aging process itself, can cause those creases, lines, and wrinkles that we all hate so much.

Q: What is skin and what does it do?
A: Skin is the largest organ in the body. In the average person, it would cover about eighteen square feet if it were spread out and would weigh about six pounds.

Our skin has many different functions. It's a protective mechanism, shielding us from environmental stresses and from injury by germs, and through its regulation of body temperature, from extreme heat and cold. It's a sensory organ that allows us to know where we are, by touch and pressure, and it's an important part of the erogenous system, providing us with pleasurable sensations.

Skin is also part of the immune system, helping to fight infections; it provides structure to our soft tissues and it keeps water in by forming a barrier. When the skin is exposed to sunshine, our body, by a chemical reaction, makes its own vitamin D.

Q: What is skin composed of and how is it structured?
A: Skin is mostly composed of protein, but it also contains a lot of fluid, collagen (a protein), and elastin fiber. The collagen, with its elastin fiber, helps our skin to "fit tight" and to return to its normal shape after it's been stretched out. But as we will see, when collagen is damaged, as can happen over time, the skin loses its elasticity, and this becomes one of the causes of wrinkles.

The outermost layer of the skin is mainly dead cells that are just piled up, similar to shingles on a roof. Normally, they come off naturally or when we dry ourselves with a towel after bathing. Beneath this is the epidermis, a thin layer that is the skin you see and the skin that shows the signs of aging.

The deepest portion of the epidermis is called the basal layer. It's the living layer where the cells grow. At the basal layer, new skin cells are born and grow upward through the epidermis until they reach the top layer, where they have now gone through their life cycle and pile up like shingles.

It takes between thirty and forty-five days for a basal cell to regenerate itself and go through one of these cycles. When you are young, the dead cells on the surface are quickly shed, but as you grow older, they can remain and accumulate, creating a dry, wrinkled skin surface.

Q: What about glands and other components in the skin?
A: The dermis, the layer of skin located beneath the epidermis, provides a cushioning support for the epidermis. That's where our sweat glands are located, which help regulate body temperature. It's also the location of hair follicles, which grow new hair; sebaceous glands or oil glands that provide natural moisturizers to the skin; and nerve endings for sensation, vibration, temperature, and pressure.

Q: What about the muscles in the skin?
A: There are some muscles in the dermis, although they are not the muscles that we treat when we inject Botox. They include goose-pimple muscles that attach to the hair follicle base and contract when we get cold.

Q: What keeps the skin supple and elastic, and what happens to make it less supple, resulting in signs of aging?
A: The two main factors are the changes in elastin fibers in the dermis and in the ground substance, which is the fluid in our skin that acts as a cushion. But aging has multiple causes, and loss of elasticity is only one of the factors involved in it.

We age chronologically and we also "photo-age," because of the effects of long-term sun exposure. You can take some eighty-year-old people and you might see less aged skin on their faces than on some thirty-five-year-olds. The eighty-year-old might have a skin type that is more naturally resistant to sun exposure, and maybe the thirty-five-year-old is fair-skinned, grew up in Los Angeles, and worked as a lifeguard, creating heavily sun-damaged skin. Many different things can contribute to the aged appearance of the skin, including nutritional factors, smoking, and rare congenital diseases, where enzyme deficiencies allow the sun to damage the skin more readily.

Q: What are the effects of chronological aging?
A: In every decade of your life, the effects of aging on the skin increase. But it's around the time when we're in our forties that the skin really starts to lose some of its elasticity. The elastic fibers tend to diminish in strength, collagen production decreases, and cellular turnover of the epidermis takes longer.

So as we get older, the protective mechanisms in our skin are weakened and DNA is damaged, whether by time or mutation, which can create more problems. There may be wrinkles, a more aged appearance on the skin's surface, or the formation of skin cancers. Less collagen creates a thinning in the dermis, so the skin becomes more transparent and we see the blood vessels on the hands more. We lose fat tissue and the dermis thins dramatically.

On the epidermis, there is much less cellular turnover, so we're not regenerating new skin as quickly, we're not replenishing ourselves, and the stressed cells don't have a chance to leave since they are not being replaced as quickly.

Q: Is the natural aging process the main cause of all these changes?

A: Believe it or not, the aged appearance of the skin is almost completely sun-induced. Studies show that as much as 95 percent of an aged appearance on the face can be traced to sun exposure.

If you take people with wrinkles on their faces who have had a lot of sun exposure, and you look at their upper inner arms or groin areas or other areas that have not been exposed to sunlight, you will typically not see the sallow color or the cobblestoning or cross-hatching of the facial skin, and you will not see the lack of elasticity as much as you will see it on the sun-exposed surfaces.

Fortunately, a vitamin-A cream, tretinoin (Retin-A), has been proven to reverse some signs of photo-damage, both visually and microscopically (see chapter 8).

Q: What about free radicals? What are they and how do they damage the skin?

A: Free radicals are molecules that contain at least one unpaired electron, causing them to bump other electrons out of orbit as they search for a pair. In large numbers, these unbalanced molecules can cause chain reactions, seriously damaging the DNA and collagen in our cells. In fact, many experts believe that free radicals are one of the major causes of premature aging.

Free radicals can be caused by illness, chemical pollution, and toxins such as tobacco smoke, poor diet, overexposure to the sun, and excessive exercise, especially in people who are not used to it, such as weekend athletes.

In proper amounts, antioxidants such as vitamin C and vitamin E can neutralize free radicals and counteract cellular damage, helping to prevent illnesses, including cancer, and the signs of aging that we all want to avoid.

Q: What do studies tell us about the signs of aging according to our chronological age?
A: They indicate that by about the age of sixty, we have lost about 50 percent of our skin's elasticity, particularly of the skin on the face. So you have a thinning of the foundation, less protein, less fluids, less cushion, less fat below that, and less elasticity. The result is "crepelike" skin that has wrinkles and doesn't snap back into position. It also has more visible understructures, such as veins. You can even have skin that eventually shears right off, peeling away with just a slight bump against a doorway, for example. And almost all of this skin is heavily sun-exposed.

Q: So sun exposure is really the crucial factor?
A: Yes. I've had patients in their seventies and eighties who have many bruises on their arms because ultraviolet rays—the deeper-penetrating rays of the sun—have damaged their collagen. Collagen is an important substance that wraps around the blood vessel wall, providing strength to blood vessels.

Not only do these people lose their skin's foundation, they also have loss around the foundation, affecting their circulation, for example. So all they need is a light touch and the blood vessel can rupture. Meanwhile, if you look at their inner forearms, there are hardly any bruises, because that part of the skin does not have a long history of sun exposure.

The bottom line is this: Sun-exposed skin ages much more severely and much more rapidly than protected skin.

Q: In addition to the sun and the natural effects of the aging process, what other factors can have an adverse effect on the appearance of the skin?
A: Both alcohol and smoking. And not only cigarette smoking, but breathing secondhand smoke as well, because smoke depletes the body of oxygen.

If you try to metabolize anything in the body with a lack of oxygen, you develop toxins. That's why people get cramps when their body does not have sufficient oxygen in one particular area.

And everyone exposed to smoke, whether from cigarettes, cigars, pipes, or secondhand smoke, is at risk of significant free-radical damage. In addition, people who are smokers and also consume alcohol and and are exposed to the sun experience a "synergistic" effect, the multiple number of causes leading to an aged appearance at a surprisingly early age.

Q: What about the effects of diet and liquid consumption on the skin?
A: If someone is deficient in essential factors, such as protein, they will have a problem. Vitamin and mineral supplements usually can't make up the difference if your overall diet is poor. You also need to be well hydrated to

make your kidneys function well and to have the "turgor," or normal fullness of the skin, which gives the skin its bounciness and firmness (see chapter 9).

When women go through their menstrual cycles or menopause, they have not only hormonal changes but also fluid changes. And having less fluid in the skin can make a big difference in terms of an aging appearance. You can compare it to a plant that isn't watered enough. The leaves droop and begin to dry out. But once you water it, the plant's leaves perk up and become stronger and fuller. Well, the skin acts in the same way.

Q: Does a dry atmosphere due to weather conditions, heating systems in winter, or air-conditioning in summer have a bad effect on the skin?
A: Definitely. You have not only a lack of moisture because of the dryness and the addition of heat in the summer, but you are also traumatizing the skin by the heat itself.

There's a similar effect from flying. People who fly a lot, such as flight attendants, often see a change in their complexions. When you're up in altitude, there is less barometric pressure, so the pressure on the skin is greater than in the air, and this kind of forces out some of the water droplets in your skin. You are evaporating more, and the dryness is robbing your system. So it's crucial to always maintain good hydration if you want to have healthy, youthful skin (see chapter 9).

Q: What about bathing a lot? Can that dry out the skin?

A: Yes, it can. People say that they are concerned about hygiene, but the normal person does not need to wash more than three times a day. That might be far too much. Oil production in the skin is there purposely to protect it.

Many young people go to a dermatologist because they think their skin is too oily, but people who have inherited a good density of facial oil glands tend to develop fine lines less quickly than those who have drier skin.

So if you wash several times a day, especially with hot water and one of the more caustic or more detergent-based cleansers, you will strip away those protective oils from the skin.

Q: Why is that so bad?
A: Believe it or not, it causes the body to make more oil. The body recognizes that the oils are being stripped away by excessive cleansing and it gets busy making more. But if you keep using hot water and detergent-based cleansers, stripping away the oil, and you don't moisturize, your skin will get redder, you'll get flaking and irritation, and it can even get so bad that you get eczema. The skin becomes so damaged that when magnified, it takes on the appearance of a dry riverbed with sections that shrink away from each other, leaving polygonal cracks.

Q: Are there people with good intentions who over-treat their skin and damage it in other ways without meaning to?
A: Yes. There are people who will use alpha hydroxy acids (see chapter 8), the fruit acids that are so commonplace in many types of products, and then combine them

with exfoliating scrubs with granules or loofah sponge scrubs, and in addition, have microdermabrasion treatment with their aesthetician or physician.

The epidermis, which is there for protection, is being removed because of this overzealous combination of treatments, increasing water loss through the epidermis. These people can develop skin irritation and chronically sensitive skin, skin that becomes red very quickly with minimal perturbation, skin that itches and hurts, skin that does not regenerate well.

Q: What about the use of cleansers and moisturizers?
A: It's actually very easy to take good care of the skin without spending a lot of money. For example, the over-the-counter cleanser Cetaphil is a relatively inexpensive nonirritating product that also acts as a moisturizer.

Sunscreens are also very important, and anyone undergoing cosmetic improvement needs to protect their investment. They should be used on a daily basis. If you use makeup, apply the sunscreen first. You should also reapply sunscreens during the day, especially if you're perspiring a lot, if you're outside for a while, after you wash, and after you go swimming (see chapter 9).

Q: Do we need to begin protecting our skin when we are children?
A: Absolutely. There's no doubt that one of the best things we can do is practice preventive medicine. We know that the aged appearance of the skin, as well as skin cancer, are caused significantly by sun exposure in childhood. This aged appearance can hasten significantly and

quickly, even overnight, with sun damage, especially with the use of suntan parlors (see chapter 9).

Childhood is definitely the best time to start with sunscreens. The American Academy of Pediatrics has said that sunscreens are safe for children and that we do not want our children to be sunburned.

Q: What about facial expressions? We know that if we smile or laugh or frown a lot, lines and wrinkles will develop over time. Do people who are very facially expressive tend to have more lines and wrinkles? Is there a direct connection between the two?
A: There are people who have inherited good genes and good oil glands and have avoided a lot of sunshine. If they frown a lot, these people don't tend to get many grooves in their skin. But people who have dry skin and lots of sun exposure over the years, including many sunburns as children, tend to get long-term creases where the muscles for facial expressions move.

But you have to realize that the lines caused by the movement of muscles, such as the lines in the forehead and the crow's-feet around the eyes, are different from the lines on the middle of the cheek. Those lines in the cheek, which I refer to as cobblestoning or cross-hatching, are mainly from sun exposure, not facial expressions.

Q: When do we begin to get those lines?
A: They actually start to form in your thirties—they begin that early. The lines on the rest of the face can start in the thirties as well. That's when we first start to see very fine creases developing around the eyes. With each de-

cade, we see more lines, moving south. We're not yet talking about the smile folds or the jowls that start to sag because of a lack of elastin and collagen support and the gravitational effect of the years.

Q: What else is happening in the skin to cause aging?
A: The fatty layer underneath the foundation starts to thin or atrophy. That causes things to shift and the skin begins to sag and droop, since it is losing its structure.

Q: Why do some people accept these lines and wrinkles that come with age, even enjoying them as "signs of character," while others are horrified and will do almost anything to get rid of them?
A: People are like snowflakes, no two alike. Everyone's actions and reactions are based on the way they were reared, environmental influences, and inherited factors. And people can suddenly change their views, too.

It's not unusual for people to come to me and say, "I never thought I'd want cosmetic surgery, but I see my friends who have had it and they've had great results. They have a different attitude and a new lease on life, and I want that, too." Or someone else might say, "I'm not doing this for myself, but I don't want to retire early and I see people around me being asked to retire because of their aged appearance."

Another might tell me, "I'm interviewing for a new job. After all these years, I was laid off, and I'd like to interview with a younger appearance. After all, people are prejudiced and they think I will be smarter and more productive if I look younger."

And someone else may say, "My significant other just broke up with me and I want to feel better about myself," or "I'm divorced and I'm seeing things on my face now that I didn't see before. I'm concerned about what someone new is going to think about me."

People have all kinds of reasons for wanting to improve their appearance. But yes, there are also many people who are content with their lines and wrinkles just the way they are.

Q: Do you ever see those people in your practice?
A: Yes. They may come in for other treatments, like removal of a skin cancer and reconstruction afterward. They may say about the treatment, which includes local anesthetic, "People go through all this just for a better appearance? I can't imagine why!"

But later on, some of these people are so pleased by the results of the skin cancer treatment that they actually change their minds and decide to have cosmetic procedures to further improve their faces. So people have many different views, and some of them will change the views they have held for many years, while others will not.

Q: Are there people who are fixated on their skin and imagine signs of aging that really aren't there?
A: Yes, this does occur. Often they are having some kind of personal problem. They think that if they can get a handle and fix something on their face, even if it's not there, they will be able to fix their real problem as well.

For example, they may want to restore the interest of

a disinterested partner or they may be unhappy with their career or have other personal difficulties.

Q: What do you do when someone like that comes to see you?
A: Physicians have to determine who is an appropriate candidate for any given treatment. They have to be certain that the patient is there for the right reason, that they actually need the treatment, and that the treatment has a good chance of being effective.

So if I see someone for a consultation who says, "Look at those lines," and I really don't see anything there or I see something very minimal, or think they won't be satisfied with the amount of improvement we can reasonably expect, I tell them they should not have treatment. I don't believe you should proceed with any treatment unless the patient and the physician are on the same wavelength. The advantages must outweigh the risks and be worth the cost.

Q: In your practice, what are the approximate percentages of women and men that you see?
A: Most of my patients are women. But in the past ten years, the number of male patients has definitely gone up. Right now, my cosmetic practice is composed of about 85 percent women and 15 percent men. The women come mainly for Botox, chemical peels, collagen injections, fat injections, noninvasive laser rejuvenation, and powered tumescent liposuction. The men come mainly for liposuction around the "love handles," but more are coming now for Botox and chemical peels. With all the recent public-

ity, I expect to see many more men coming in for Botox treatments.

To Summarize:

- Skin is the largest organ in the body and has multiple functions.

- Skin is composed of protein and fluids, including collagen and elastin fiber, which help keep it tight and young looking.

- Aging skin does not shed surface dead cells as efficiently, creating a dry, wrinkled surface.

- Loss of collagen and elasticity in the skin creates signs of aging.

- Long-term sun exposure is the single most important factor in the creation of aged skin.

- Free radicals in the body can damage skin; antioxidants, such as vitamins C and E, can counteract them. Vitamin A creams (tretinoin) can reverse some signs of photo-damage, both visually and microscopically.

- Heavy smoking and alcohol consumption seriously damage skin, making it look much older.

- A well-balanced diet, with sufficient protein and good fluid intake, is important for healthy skin.

- Skin must be kept well hydrated. Too much bathing and washing can cause dry or irritated skin.

- Lines on the face begin to form in the thirties and increase with each decade.

- Always use sunscreen and moisturizers regularly.

Chapter 2

What Is Botox and How Can It Rejuvenate Your Skin?

We have seen how the skin ages, forming lines, wrinkles, and creases on your face, making you look much older and less attractive than you want to look. Although you can improve your skin through better care, including protecting it from further damage, you cannot restore your youthful appearance or make any major improvements without some kind of medical treatment.

Until the appearance of Botox, most treatments for skin rejuvenation involved either major surgery or potential problems with unwanted side effects (see chapter 8).

Without a doubt, Botox is revolutionary: an inexpensive, rapid, minimally invasive procedure that can literally take years off your face. Let's find out exactly what it is, how it was developed, and how it works its miracles.

Q: What is Botox? What is in that little bottle and how is it made in the laboratory?
A: Botox is a purified protein, a diluted form of the botulinum toxin, which, in its concentrated form, causes the potentially deadly disease botulism. It is produced from fermentation of the Hall strain of *Clostridium botulinum* type-A toxin, sterilized and vacuum-dried in the laboratory, and grown in a medium containing casein hydrolysate, glucose, and yeast extract.

Botox is sold in bottles or vials containing 100 units. It is kept in a freezer in the doctor's office and is reconstituted with saline solution before being injected.

Q: But the toxin that causes botulism is so dangerous. How can Botox be safe?
A: It is not a practical concern because the amount of the botulinum toxin in Botox is known to be well within the safe limit.

Any toxic chemical is only toxic at a certain level. For example, the local anesthetic lidocaine that we get in the dentist's office could kill us if it were given in a much higher concentration. Even aspirin can kill at a toxic level. So almost any chemical in a concentrated form has the potential for being fatal.

In order for a product to be approved by the FDA, the parameters must be documented by the researchers and the safe levels versus the toxic doses for administration proven. The Botox dose that we use for reversing signs of aging skin is extremely small and well within the safe level. In addition, according to the manufacturer Allergan, the toxin is broken down and leaves the body within twenty-four to forty-eight hours, so there is no possibility of a buildup over time with continued treatments.

Botox has been used by neurologists for decades in much higher doses than we use for skin treatments. Neurologists may use 400 units in a session, and we use only 30 to 100 units on average. Yet there has not been one single case of botulism created by any of these injections.

And now millions of people have been injected with Botox, the number one cosmetic medical treatment. The studies show that there are very few side effects and that it is a remarkably safe drug.

Q: Can you tell us a little about the history of Botox? How was it discovered and what were its uses in the past?
A: The actual bacterium, *Bacillus botulinus,* was identified in 1895 by a Belgian researcher. It was purified in crystalline form in 1946 by Dr. Edward Schantz. In the 1970s, Dr. Schantz, working with Dr. Alan Scott of the Smith-Kettlewell Eye Research Foundation, discovered that the toxin, botulinum toxin A, corrected crossed eyes in laboratory monkeys. A few years later, Dr. Scott began to test the toxin's effectiveness in treating muscle spasms around the eyes of humans.

But the real breakthrough came in 1987, when Dr. Jean Carruthers, a Canadian ophthalmologist, noticed that after she used the drug to treat eye muscle spasms, the crow's-feet lines around the eyes of her patients improved dramatically. When she mentioned this side effect to her husband, dermatologist Alastair Carruthers, he decided to try it out on his receptionist. And that was how we discovered that the drug now known as Botox can reverse some of the signs of aging on the face.

Q: When was Botox actually approved by the FDA?
A: The FDA approved Botox for treating strabismus, or lazy eye (see below), in 1989.

Q: What does Botox actually do to achieve its results?
A: Botox works locally, not systemically. That means that if we inject it into the forehead, it only affects the forehead, not the muscles in the foot. It remains in the area where it's injected.

When the muscles contract to make creases in the skin, they require nerves to provide their stimulus from the brain to the muscle. The nerve does that by promoting an electric signal, which liberates a chemical called a neurotransmitter. The neurotransmitter sends the signal between the nerves and also between the nerves and other structures, such as muscles.

The specific neurotransmitter involved with Botox is acetylcholine, which is released from the end of the nerves to the receptor in the muscle. The brain makes a signal and the nerve releases the acetylcholine, which stimulates the muscle to contract. But if the receptor is blocked, the muscle doesn't receive the signal.

Botox blocks acetylcholine from making that connection, and as a result, the muscle is unable to contract. Since the muscle can't contract, the skin on the face is unable to form the unwanted lines, wrinkles, or creases. In effect, the muscle is paralyzed, and the lines, wrinkles, and creases diminish or disappear.

Q: Prior to its cosmetic use on the skin, what were some of the medical conditions that Botox had been used to treat?
A: Botox has been useful for a wide range of medical problems and is still used to treat them. Other possible uses are also being studied.

Botox has been FDA approved to treat cervical dystonia, which is a condition involving involuntary contractions or spasms of the neck muscles. An example is wryneck (torticollis), a condition of painful muscle contractions that distort the neck. If this condition is not relieved by other treatment, Botox can often be used successfully.

Also, patients with muscular dystrophy or a stroke, for example, often develop muscular spasms of the neck because they are unable to move for a long time. By injecting Botox, these neck spasms can be eased. Botox can also help to restore equality between one side of the head and the other when one side has been significantly weakened.

Ophthalmologists use Botox for a condition called blepharospasm, which is uncontrollable, exaggerated, and tight closure of their eyelids, causing the eyelids to squint or even close shut altogether. Sometimes patients will blink so hard that their eyebrows come all the way down, and of course, they can't control it. This condition can also cause headaches and loss of sleep. Botox injections can relax the muscles that cause this involuntary blinking and often get rid of the problem. Botox has FDA approval for use in treating blepharospasm.

Botox has also been useful in treating strabismus, a medical condition in which the eyes are misaligned and point in different directions. This condition is also called "lazy eye," and it can cause serious problems with vision, including an inability to perceive depth, vision loss, and even functional blindness. With Botox, the eye muscles responsible for this condition may relax, and in some cases surgery can be avoided. Botox has FDA approval for this use.

Excessive sweating is another condition that responds well to Botox. Most people don't realize how disabling this condition can be for those who suffer from it. If someone is perspiring excessively, it's not unusual for them to be standing there, sweat literally dripping off their fingers onto the floor, creating a puddle. Their shoes are ruined and have to be replaced, their shirts are ruined, and they are often socially embarrassed. They can't get through job interviews, shake hands, or appear in public. And sometimes they perspire excessively even when they are completely calm.

Botox injections under the arms, in the palms, and in the soles of the feet can often greatly diminish this problem.

Another condition Botox seems to help is migraine headaches. In fact Allergan, the manufacturer of Botox, has applied to the FDA for approval of Botox to treat migraines. (Note: Physicians are legally permitted to use an FDA-approved drug for any medical purpose they find warranted, even though the FDA has not specifically approved it for that use. This is called "off-label" use and it is very common and medically ethical.) Although the exact causes of migraines remain unknown, studies show that a significant percentage of migraine patients improve with Botox injections. That would seem to lead to the conclusion that muscle tension and spasms are connected with at least some cases of chronic migraines.

Botox is also used to treat back pain, which is frequently linked to muscle spasms around the spine. According to one study, 63 percent of patients who received Botox treatment said that their back pain was reduced by at least 50 percent.

Spasmodic dysphonia is another condition that responds well to Botox. It is characterized by muscle spasms and tightness affecting the vocal cords, causing the voice to become strained and hoarse. Before Botox, surgery was the only effective treatment.

Finally, giving Botox to children with cerebral palsy can help preserve their range of motion and, in some cases, help them avoid the need for braces or surgery.

Botox is also being studied for possible use in treating Parkinson's disease and Tourette's syndrome.

Q: Is Botox completely safe for all these uses, including cosmetic uses on the face?
A: There are patients who have used it medically for over twenty years and cosmetically for about fifteen years, and from all the evidence we have, it appears to be very safe. In addition, over these years of use there have not been any incidents of concern and no long-term dangerous side effects that have been directly connected to the use of Botox.

But it is impossible to guarantee that we won't learn something negative in the coming years. So we advise patients to maintain an ongoing dialogue with their physicians so that if anything new is discovered, they will be informed.

Q: Why does Botox treatment have to be repeated after only a few months? Where does the Botox go after it has been injected and why do the effects wear off?
A: Allergan, the manufacturer of Botox, has stated that the protein from the botulinum toxin A that is the active ingredient in Botox breaks down and leaves the body within twenty-four to forty-eight hours of being injected. But the effects of temporarily paralyzing the muscle last for three or four months, because the Botox has temporarily disconnected the nerve's ability to communicate with the muscle by disrupting the release of the chemical acetylcholine, the neurotransmitter that we mentioned before. It takes three or four months, and sometimes longer, for the nerve to reconnect to the muscle, and that's when another Botox treatment is needed.

So the diluted botulinum toxin A is excreted from the body within forty-eight hours and there is no possibility of any kind of buildup in the body with further treatments. But because acetylcholine release has been disrupted, there is a gradual return to the former state that existed before the Botox shot was given.

Q: What happens if you don't go back and get more Botox treatments after the effects wear off? Does the skin go back to the way it was or does it get worse?
A: No, it never gets worse, but there are patients who have actually been able to break their habits of scrunching up their faces or raising their brows or frowning continually, and this can help them to minimize the creases and lines.

Other than this, and all other things being equal, once

the Botox has worn off, the same lines and wrinkles will return to the skin if the injections are not continued.

Q: Is it possible to use too much Botox, and if so, what can happen?
A: The theory is that if you use too much, you can create a stimulus for the body to create antibodies to counter its effect. So if you give Botox in too high a dose or repeat the injections too often, you're really asking your body to defend against it and you may not get the nice effect you want. The added Botox injections will not be able to work in the body and you may end up paying money for nothing. That's one important reason why you want to stick to the injection schedule recommended by your physician, even though this effect has not been shown to occur so far with cosmetic Botox use.

There are also some people who think that since Botox is so effective, greater amounts will be better. They may go to different physicians to get more than the recommended doses, and some of these people can wind up with more muscles paralyzed than they really want, giving them frozen or expressionless faces. Of course these effects will wear off with time, but you really have to be careful to use only the amount you actually need. In fact, responsible physicians will always use the minimum amount of Botox to get the desired effect.

Q: Can Botox be used to prevent lines and wrinkles from forming?
A: Yes. If I had patients who were interested in doing that, I would go ahead and inject them, but I don't nor-

mally propose that kind of treatment myself.

One of the reasons is that it's easy enough to treat the lines once they have formed and I don't like doing treatments that don't seem necessary. But if a patient came to me and said, "My mother has terrible lines and I have every single feature of my mother and am certain I'm going to develop those lines, too," then I would consider Botox treatment as preventive. I would certainly check the muscle movements to see if they would create the lines the person is worrying about before embarking on treatment.

There is also a cost issue here, and patients have to be certain that they want to invest their money for a treatment that might not be necessary. And of course, if they do go ahead with preventive treatment, I will be certain that they take all the recommended precautions to avoid damaging their skin, such as regular use of sunscreen.

Q: Is Botox really a miracle drug? Is it significantly better than previous treatments for aging skin?
A: It may not be a true miracle, but I can say that we don't have any other treatment that is such an effective muscle relaxer for cosmetic uses. Everything that we were doing prior to Botox was filling and sanding and pulling. So Botox gives us a totally different approach.

For example, there is surgery to improve the deep crease between the eyebrows. Surgeons go in and make a very big cut, from temple to temple, across the hairline, high on the forehead and forward scalp. As a result, some patients get numbness of the scalp and they may also have a long, visible scar. To minimize this, surgeons now go in endoscopically with long catheters and make small incisions to cut the muscles between the eyebrows.

The effect is more long-term than Botox, but it's also not always permanent because the muscle can reattach or regrow. Botox can do a very good job of improving that crease between the eyebrows, and do it quickly, with minimal risk and without any surgery.

Compared with collagen injections for deep creases between the eyes, Botox is certainly much better. When it comes to eyelid creases and crow's-feet, collagen can bead under the thin skin, making it look like little pebbles along the skin's surface (see chapter 8). But Botox will give you a smoothing effect without any beading. So Botox is quite an advance over many previous treatments.

Q: The cosmetic use of Botox is approved by the FDA for treating the creases between the eyebrows, also called glabellar lines. What other conditions is Allergan now studying in anticipation of applying for future specific FDA approvals?
A: Botox is being studied for future FDA-approved use for treating crow's-feet lines, forehead lines, chronic tension headaches, migraines, hyperhidrosis (extreme sweating), upper-limb spasticity (excessive muscle contraction), and juvenile cerebral palsy.

Q: What do you see for the future of Botox? Will there be new and better drugs before long or will Botox remain a major treatment for some time?
A: I think Botox is here to stay. Other brands have been manufactured, but the theory behind its use will be around for quite some time. Botox will never be the only treat-

ment for these conditions, but it will remain an effective choice for many patients, and a wonderful adjunct to other cosmetic treatments.

To Summarize:

- Botox is a highly diluted, purified form of botulinum toxin A.

- Botox is not toxic and has been found quite safe with very few side effects. The toxin leaves the body twenty-four to forty-eight hours after injection.

- Not one single case of botulism has ever resulted from the medical use of Botox in over twenty years, or the cosmetic use of Botox in over fifteen years; millions of patients have been treated.

- Botox was first used to treat facial lines in 1987 by Dr. Alastair Carruthers.

- Botox is injected into muscles and works only in those muscles. It blocks the release of the neurotransmitter acetylcholine, temporarily paralyzing muscles that create facial lines, creases, and wrinkles. These lines then fade or disappear.

- Botox is also used to treat many different medical conditions.

- Botox treatments must be repeated every three to six months in order to maintain their effect.

- Without further Botox treatments, the skin will return to its previous state after a few months.

- Too much Botox can cause antibodies to form, making it ineffective. It can also cause a "frozen" or expressionless face. Stick to your doctor's recommended schedule.

- Botox can be used to prevent lines from ever forming.

- Botox is the most effective treatment of its kind for minimizing facial lines and restoring a more youthful appearance.

Chapter 3

Is Botox Right for You?

You now understand what Botox is, how it works, and some of the things it can do. But is it right for you? There are some people who should not use Botox—are you one of them? In addition, there are other factors to consider before deciding if you want to try this treatment or continue if you are already using it. In this chapter, we will examine some of those issues and help guide you to a decision about whether or not to proceed.

Q: Are there people who should not use Botox?
A: Anyone who has an allergy to any component that's included in Botox should not use it, of course. One of those ingredients is albumin, a type of protein derived from human blood. Botox is grown in a medium containing casein hydrolysate, glucose, and yeast extract and is dissolved in a sterile sodium chloride solution containing

human albumin before it is sterile-filtered and vacuum-dried. I'm not aware of anyone who has had an allergic reaction to the product, but it is a possibility, and if you think you may be allergic to any of these substances, you should inform your physician before using Botox.

It is also theoretically possible for the albumin to contain infectious material linked to diseases, such as Creutzfeldt-Jacob disease, but there has never been a case of any viral infection being transmitted by the human albumin in Botox. This albumin is carefully screened by the laboratory prior to use in Botox.

There are also some medications that can interact badly with Botox. An example are aminoglycosides, antibiotic medications that can affect the kidneys. If someone is using Botox, it is possible that the Botox can affect the level of aminoglycosides so that the patient could suddenly have a dangerously high level. So if you are on this kind of medication, you should not use Botox.

There are a few other medications that should not be combined with Botox, including lincosamides, polymyxins, quinidine, magnesium sulfate, anticholinesterases, and succinylcholine chloride.

Botox should also not be used by women who are pregnant or breast-feeding or who are thinking about getting pregnant.

Q: Is there any evidence that Botox can harm the fetus or newborn?
A: Not at this time, because the studies have not yet been done. In medicine, we are always concerned about potential effects on a fetus or growing baby, so when we don't know, we are very conservative. But so far, there is no

scientific evidence that Botox is harmful to a developing fetus or to newborns through transmission in breast milk.

There is a case on record of a woman who canned her own vegetables, didn't do it properly, and then got botulism from eating the contaminated vegetables. She was pregnant, and while she had some of the symptoms of botulism, such as impaired breathing, she recovered, and there was no harm to her baby, who was born healthy.

Q: Do people with certain medical conditions have to avoid Botox?
A: There are some neurological conditions that require caution with Botox. One example is myasthenia gravis. Some patients who suffer from this disease have droopy eyelids that get worse during the course of the day—they are usually more severe at night. Botox could aggravate this problem. Another condition, Horner's syndrome, also frequently involves droopy eyelids.

Other medical problems, such as muscular dystrophy, double vision, easy bleeding, Parkinson's disease, and past surgeries, could make Botox an unwise choice. Every potential Botox patient is asked for a complete medical history (see chapter 5) and each one is individually evaluated in order to determine if Botox is safe for that person.

In addition, anyone who has an infection or inflammatory skin problem, such as eczema, psoriasis, or skin allergic contact dermatitis, at the site where Botox will be injected can't proceed with the treatment until the skin clears up completely.

Allergan, the manufacturer of Botox, also cautions physicians about using Botox with people over the age of sixty-five, since studies on this age group have not been completed. There is no scientific evidence that Botox is dangerous in any way for people over sixty-five, but its safety has not been proven yet.

Physicians should be cautious when treating this population for forehead wrinkles, as they may already have droopy foreheads, which Botox can accentuate, leading to lower eyelids that can obstruct upper visual fields.

Q: What about children?
A: Again, because it has not been scientifically proven safe for this age group and because children have significant physical differences from adults, cosmetic Botox is not recommended for anyone under the age of eighteen. However, Botox is used by neurologists for treating children who have some of the medical problems we already mentioned, such as cerebral palsy.

Q: Are there any people who should not use Botox for psychological reasons?
A: Emotionally stable people seem to benefit from Botox. People who are mentally ill may not be able to give informed consent to treatment, so they should not be treated. In an extreme case, if someone was suicidal and said something like, "I must have Botox, and if it doesn't work, I'll kill myself," a responsible physician would not want to provide Botox treatment. Psychological treatment would have to come first.

But if people are emotionally healthy and well balanced, Botox treatment appears to have only positive effects. The doctor just has to make sure that the patient wants the treatment for the right reason. Botox will not fix emotional problems, it will just make you look better and perhaps feel better about yourself.

Q: What do patients tell you that lets you know they are good candidates for Botox?
A: When I ask them why they want to use Botox on their frown lines, for instance, they will say, "I want to get rid of this crease so I will look younger and feel better." If they say, "I want this because my boyfriend or my husband doesn't like it and he told me to get rid of it," I might discuss it with them a little more.

Q: Does any previous cosmetic surgery or other skin treatment have any effect on the results you will get with Botox? Do people who have had plastic surgery or collagen injections get better results or does it make no difference?
A: Previous surgery or cosmetic treatments have no relationship to whether or not Botox is appropriate and they don't affect your Botox results. But there are certain physical characteristics that can influence Botox treatment.

For example, as some people age they develop a forehead that droops, with their eyebrows coming down lower than they used to be. Since the eyebrow actually helps to hold up the eyelid, these people often move their muscles to raise their eyebrows so they can see better.

So let's say we use Botox on the forehead of such people. They won't be able to use their forehead to keep their eyelids up. For several weeks or even months after the injections, they may get eyelid lowering, an effect they definitely do not want. So before we administer Botox to the forehead, we have to find out who is a good candidate, and someone with a preexisting forehead droop is at higher risk for unwanted side effects.

Q: Is it possible to get a good idea of how Botox will work for you by looking at your friends' results? Or are results unique to each individual?
A: The results you get with Botox are always unique. There is a spectrum of change and the lines on one person's face are always slightly different from the lines on someone else's face. Your friends may have deeper lines or lines that are a bit farther away from the eyelid area or a bit closer, so your effect will be different.

And everyone's muscles are different. Some people have very strong, big-bellied muscles in the forehead or between the eyebrows or around the crow's-feet. There are people who not only wrinkle around the eyes because of constant squinting, but who also have a very big smile. If your friend has two sets of muscles that created a line, but yours are a result of just one set of muscles, your results can be quite different and probably better than your friend's.

Q: Although the manufacturer of Botox has not endorsed treatment for people over the age of sixty-five, the physician can still decide to treat such people. What is your opinion about Botox for people over sixty-five?
A: For older people, we know that metabolism often decreases, the liver is less efficient, and certain medications should be lower in dose than those given to younger

people. And because no studies have been done in this age group, I think physicians should be conservative when treating anyone over the age of sixty-five with Botox.

Q: What lines and wrinkles are most commonly treated by Botox?
A: There are three major areas of the face that are most often treated: (1) the furrow or frown lines between the brows, also called the glabellar lines, which are controlled by the corrugator, procerus, and orbicularis muscles; (2) the horizontal lines on the forehead, which are controlled by the frontalis muscles; (3) the crow's-feet lines around the eyes, which are controlled by the orbicularis oculi muscles. The FDA has given Allergan approval for Botox to treat only the glabellar lines, but the company will be seeking approval for the other two areas at some time in the future.

Botox can also be used for certain lines in the neck and on a few other places on the face, which we will discuss shortly.

Q: What lines and wrinkles are usually not treated by Botox?
A: It's very important to know that Botox is typically not used around the mouth. That means it is not effective for the smile folds that bother so many people. These lines are not muscle wrinkles, although there is a possibility that in the future, a way to use Botox on them might be developed.

Botox is also not used on the horizontal crease that some people have on the lower eyelid, in the middle, underneath the pupil. But it can be used on the side of the eye and also on the neck, in the areas where muscles contract.

And in the past few months, I've had inquiries from patients about the crosshatch wrinkles in the middle of the cheek, but again, these are not treated by Botox because they are sun-related, not muscle-related.

Q: Aside from the three major areas of the face that are most often treated by Botox—forehead lines, frown lines between the eyebrows, and crows'-feet around the eyes—what other areas will respond to Botox?

A: Botox can be used to improve dimpling in the chin and grooves that form in the corner of the lower lip when we age. We can put a little Botox in the muscle of the lower lip corners and it may help lift them up, creating a younger appearance by lessening the sagging and minimizing the creases.

There are also some areas on the neck that can be treated with Botox. The neck has both transverse (horizontal) creases in some people and turkey-gobbler bands in other people, and both of these can be improved by Botox. Botox treatment for the latter never gets as good a result as having a surgical treatment, but many people simply do not want to go under the knife, and Botox is a good alternative.

Q: Are there people with whom potential patients can talk in order to help them decide if they want to proceed?

A: If you have friends or relatives who have used Botox, they can be a wonderful source of information. If you make an appointment with a physician, his or her office staff, including nurses and receptionists, can often tell you about the treatment, since they have seen so many patients and may have been treated with Botox themselves.

Sometimes people may ask for a referral to a patient who has had Botox treatment, but they are usually satisfied talking to the nurses and office staff, and to their friends.

Q: One important consideration for many people is the cost of Botox treatment. Since the injections have to be repeated every few months in order to maintain the effect, the cost can be rather high over time. About how much does an average Botox treatment cost and is there ever any insurance coverage?

A: The cost of a Botox treatment is going to vary according to the physician you choose and your geographical area, as well as what specific type of treatment you have and how much Botox is required for your procedure(s) (see chapter 6). But we can estimate the average cost as between $350 and $1,000 per treatment and the frequency as about three times a year. Whether you can afford it or whether you want to spend the money is of course entirely up to you. Health insurance does not cover the cosmetic use of Botox, and I'm not aware that it even covers medical uses, such as treatment for migraines. Patients should check with their insurance companies first if this is a concern.

Q: Why do some people want treatments and others do not?

A: I find that most people want to look better and they feel better when they like what they see in the mirror. In most cases, it's not vanity, just a desire to be their best.

When cosmetic treatments work well, people report that they are happier in their lives, more relaxed, and have more pleasant interactions at work and in their private lives. There seems to be an effect that goes far beyond just their physical looks.

But there are other people who are happy with their looks, including their wrinkles and lines, and are not self-conscious or concerned about looking youthful. There are many reasons for these differences.

As a consequence, each person has to decide individually what she or he wants to do. One wonderful aspect of Botox is that the effects wear off in a few months. So if people decide to give it a try and they're not happy for any reason, in a few short months, they can go right back to how they looked before.

SOME QUESTIONS TO ASK YOURSELF WHEN DECIDING WHETHER TO TRY BOTOX

☐ Why do I want to use Botox? Exactly what do I want to accomplish?

☐ What physical effects do I expect to achieve? Which lines and creases do I want to minimize or get rid of and why?

☐ Am I certain that Botox is an appropriate treatment for these specific problems?

☐ Can I afford to keep up the treatment if I want to?

☐ Do I have any of the conditions that indicate I should not use Botox (allergies, pregnancy or desire to get pregnant, breast-feeding, medications that interact adversely with Botox, neurological diseases, bleeding easily, double vision, dystrophy, myalgias)?

☐ Do I understand how Botox works and that even though it is thought to be safe, there could possibly be long-term unknown effects?

☐ Am I willing to deal with any possible side effects during or after treatment, such as bruising, pain, droopy eyelid, raised corners of the eyebrows, or drooling (see chapter 7)?

☐ Do I think that the changes in my appearance from Botox could have a major effect on my life and am I prepared for this possibility?

☐ Are my expectations unrealistic or do I think Botox will solve some or all of my personal problems?

☐ Do I want to invest the time and effort to find a good physician and try this treatment to improve my appearance?

There are no right or wrong answers to these questions. By studying your answers, you may find important clues to help you decide whether or not Botox may be right for you.

To Summarize:

- People who should not use Botox include those with allergies to its components; those taking medications such as aminoglycosides, which can interact badly; women who are pregnant, breast-feeding, or thinking about getting pregnant; and people with certain neuromuscular diseases, such as myasthenia gravis.

- Botox results are unique to each person. You don't know exactly how it will work until you try it.

- Botox is used to treat three main areas of the face: the frown lines between the brows, the horizontal lines on the forehead, and the crow's-feet lines around the eyes. It can also be used on the neck and for dimples in the chin.

- Botox is not usually used for smile folds around the mouth, the horizontal crease on the lower eyelid, or the cross-hatching or cobblestoning marks on the cheeks.

- Botox treatments can cost from $350 to $1,000 or more, depending on your geographical location, your doctor, and how many injections you need. Insurance coverage is not available.

• Botox will wear off in a few months, so if you don't like your results, there is no need to worry.

Chapter 4

How Can You Find the Right Doctor?

By now, you should have a pretty good idea about whether or not you are interested in trying Botox treatment. If you think you are a good candidate and want to pursue it, your next step will be to find a good doctor. In this chapter, we will guide you to the people and organizations that can be of help. You will learn who is qualified to administer Botox and how to find the doctor who is right for you.

Q: Which medical professionals are qualified to do Botox treatments? Can dentists, nurses, or just anybody provide Botox injections? Are there any laws or regulations governing its use?

A: If you want to be safe, you should receive Botox injections only from licensed physicians who have some special training and expertise in its use.

As we have seen, Botox can be used to treat a variety of medical conditions and to treat cosmetic problems, mainly in three areas on the face.

While it is certainly legal for any licensed physician to administer Botox, a patient should seek out a doctor who has been trained in its use, has experience treating patients with Botox, and has a specialty in a related field. So I would strongly recommend that if you want Botox treatment, you see, first and foremost, a board-certified dermatologist, plastic surgeon, ophthalmologist, or ENT (eye, nose, and throat) facial plastic surgeon.

Q: Why do doctors need special training?
A: Because there is a great deal to know about using Botox. Doctors need to assess each patient and make judgments about whether to inject, how much to inject, where to inject, how often to inject, and how to handle any problems that might arise. It's a complex technique that requires special training and a lot of actual experience with patients. And most of the medical professionals being trained with Botox today practice one of the specialties listed above.

Q: How can someone find a good doctor for Botox treatment?
A: The two best ways to find a doctor for anything are always a referral from your regular doctor and a recommendation from your friends who have had the treatment.

First, speak to your doctor. You may find that he or she recommends you to someone you like and you decide to go ahead with treatment. But you may also be referred to someone you don't care for, or your doctor may not know anyone to recommend for Botox.

Then you should go to your friends who have had Botox treatment. Nothing is as good as word of mouth from people who have had the treatment. They can always tell you how good a doctor is, and of course, you can see the results for yourself on their faces.

Q: What if you can't get the name of a doctor that way? What other options are available?
A: Then you have to do some research. There are some very helpful organizations you can contact for referrals (see the resources section at the end of this book). I especially like the American Society for Dermatologic Surgery because it is a subset of dermatologists who decided to concentrate on dermatologic surgery and make an effort to increase their learning in the field of cosmetic procedures.

You can also contact the people at Allergan, the manufacturer of Botox, and they will give you referrals to dermatologists, plastic surgeons, ENT facial plastic surgeons, and ophthalmologists in your area who have expertise in using Botox.

The American Academy of Cosmetic Surgery and the other organizations listed in the resources section can also provide physician referrals.

You can also look on the Internet, check the Yellow Pages or ads in newspapers and magazines, call local hospitals, and contact doctors who write articles or appear in the media talking about Botox. But your best bets remain personal recommendations from your doctor and from your friends who have used Botox and are happy with their results.

Q: You mentioned board certification. What does that mean and why is it important when selecting a doctor?
A: Doctors who are board-certified in a specific field of medicine have completed 100 percent of their training in that field. They have studied the required material and passed an examination given by the American board in their particular specialty. The board is composed of physicians in that specialty and falls under the jurisdiction of the American Board of Medical Specialties.

So if physicians are board-certified, it means they have fully completed training and have taken and passed a test administered by their peers.

Q: If physicians are not board-certified, does it mean they are not qualified in their specialty?
A: No, it does not mean that. Although such doctors are not yet finished with their specialized training, they may perform a procedure as well as someone who is board-certified. But the chances are they are not as experienced as someone who is board-certified.

You also have to remember that when a procedure first comes out, a physician in residency may be as good or better at performing it than a physician who has been practicing for twenty years. There are also physicians who are technically very good and have completed all their training, but did not pass their board exams.

So is being board-certified in itself a requirement for using Botox? No. Is it advisable? Yes, it can only help.

Q: Is it possible for potential Botox patients to talk to doctors on the phone before making an appointment so they can get more information?
A: Physicians usually do not speak to new patients on the phone prior to their coming in to the office. However, people can call and speak with a patient coordinator, if there is one in the office, or a well-informed nurse or receptionist. That way, they can get some of their questions answered.

Most doctors don't talk to prospective patients because most of the patients' questions are basic and can be answered by the staff. And it is really impossible for the doctor to answer the important questions about treatment without actually seeing the patient.

For instance, people may ask, "Am I a good candidate and will Botox help my wrinkles?" We can't answer that until we see them in the office and examine their faces.

Although it is possible for a physician to ask callers if they have a big crease between their eyebrows, we have to actually see the crease and see how much it distends when we pull it apart. In addition, we have to review prospective patients' medical histories before we can decide what treatment, if any, is appropriate.

Q: So that's why people have to come in for a consultation to answer most of their questions?
A: Yes. That's what a consultation is all about. We can

answer their questions about Botox and what it can do for them, based on their unique situation, once we have had a chance to see them and evaluate them.

Q: Do patients have to pay for a consultation or will a physician provide one without a fee?
A: That varies from doctor to doctor. There also might be group practices where one doctor will waive the consultation fee and another will not. So you really have to ask.

Q: How many doctors should you investigate or talk to before you select one? Do you need to get a second opinion before proceeding with Botox?
A: You should use your common sense regarding a second opinion, but I don't think it's usually necessary. Most of the time you don't need to see a second doctor if the doctor you see is recommended by someone you respect, and if you and the doctor seem to be on the same wavelength regarding treatment.

Q: What if you feel the doctor is pressuring you to have work done that you did not come in for?
A: A lot of physicians perform cosmetic treatment—it's sort of an art—and they have different viewpoints. There are physicians who will do only what you ask, and there are other physicians who will tell you that you look older than you should and need your whole face done.

If you're happy with yourself and the only thing you're unhappy with is the crease between your eyebrows, you should just have that done and no more. If a physician appears to be trying to persuade you to do things because they bother him or her, and they don't bother you, then you might want to see another doctor.

Q: What if you're not sure what you need?
A: That's a different story. If you say, "Doctor, I'm not sure what it is that bothers me about my face, but I want to look younger," then the doctor can ethically reply, "I would suggest a brow-lift, a face-lift, a neck-lift, fat injections for the smile creases, Botox between the eyes and for the crow's-feet around the eyes," or whatever else seems appropriate for that person.

I think you can tell when you feel comfortable with a physician and his or her recommendations. If you see a physician who has been recommended by a friend who has received treatment and is happy, or one has been referred by your regular doctor, and you like what you hear from this doctor, then you should feel comfortable going ahead with treatment.

Q: So you don't have to be quite as cautious in choosing a physician as you would, for example, if you were having major surgery?
A: Patients should be careful, but you also have to remember that Botox is a temporary, nonsurgical treatment that wears off. Don't forget that the side-effect profile with Botox is very good. So even if you have some minor side effects after treatment, they are only temporary. A Botox injection is not like having surgery, where a nerve is cut and there is no easy way to repair it.

Q: Is it important to select a doctor who has a lot of experience with Botox?
A: Yes, it is important because, again, using Botox is somewhat of an art and you want to get the most effective treatment. For instance, there are areas of the face that should not be injected, and it can take some experience to learn where they are.

Physicians who are just learning to use Botox should make this fact plain to patients—at least to the first ten patients they treat—and explain that they are just beginning and they have only recently learned the technique. Most patients will accept that. In fact, it is not uncommon for physicians doing a new procedure to initially charge reduced fees. They may also do their first procedures on employees in their office before treating regular patients.

Q: Is it difficult to use Botox properly?
A: There are some nuances with Botox. It is not something that can simply be learned by going to a one-hour conference and then starting to inject the next day. A physician needs to observe another experienced physician using Botox after studying the fundamentals.

Q: How much experience with Botox should someone look for in a doctor?
A: If a physician has been using Botox for several months and has treated many patients, that could be sufficient. But if a doctor with six months' experience is only treating one Botox patient a month, that might not be enough. A good question to ask the doctor would be how many Bo-

tox patients he or she sees in a week, and if the answer is five or ten or more, that could be a good sign.

Q: Do doctors need special training in the use of Botox?

A: It is preferable, and a patient can certainly ask the doctor about it. "How did you get your training in Botox?" Was the doctor trained during a conference? Or by watching a video on Botox? Did the doctor actually rotate with a physician already experienced with Botox and directly observe that physician using Botox?

The best-trained doctor is one who has not only read about Botox and seen videos, but has also directly observed an experienced doctor using it on patients, has then done the procedure under the direct supervision of another physician who uses Botox, and has treated a fair number of patients for at least six months.

Q: Is a consultation always a separate appointment or can you have your first Botox treatment at the same time if you want to?

A: In most cases they are combined. In the privacy of the doctor's office, if everything sounds good to the patients, if they understand all the steps in the procedure, and if the doctor feels they are good candidates, then the patient and the doctor may decide to perform the first Botox treatment at that time. In fact, about 90 percent of my patients who come for Botox consultations have their first Botox treatment during that visit.

Q: Is a "Botox party" a good way to find a doctor? Many people are going to these parties. Are they a good idea?
A: The American Academy of Dermatology has issued a statement that Botox parties are not safe, they are not a good idea, and they do not reflect the professional interests of physicians.

It is difficult to approve of Botox injections given at parties where alcohol is served and which are held in restaurants, people's homes, hotel suites, or other nonmedical settings. The environment may not be completely sanitary and there may also be safety hazards, such as those involving the disposal of used syringes.

The fact that alcohol is sometimes served at these parties is another red flag. We strongly recommend that Botox patients not drink alcoholic beverages before treatment because of the potential for bruising. In addition, if people are under the influence of *anything,* they are not truly giving their informed consent for a procedure.

In a party atmosphere, people can sometimes be coerced into doing things they would not normally do. It would be fine if the party just included a lecture and a video demonstration about Botox treatment and then the people who were interested in Botox could make an appointment and go to the doctor's office for treatment another day.

Q: Can Botox parties ever be acceptable?
A: Yes, it's possible. If the parties are held in a sterile environment where no alcohol is served and the Botox is administered by a qualified physician who remains on the

site in case any of the people have adverse reactions. If thorough consultations are done at the time, then such a seminar and treatment could be appropriate. It's also important for the physician to take care of the proper documentation, recording how many units of Botox were delivered and into which areas of each patient's face.

Q: After you gather a lot of information, how do you decide whether or not you want to go ahead and try Botox?
A: If you're still deliberating after a lot of research, the best thing to do is go in for a consultation. Learn about it, listen to the doctor's analysis of your skin problems, and then make a decision. Don't feel that you're going to be coerced into having Botox that same day if you don't want it or if you're still not certain.

There is a last step to take when you can't make up your mind: you can ask the office if there are any patients you could talk to. This is something doctors rarely do in dealing with Botox patients, but some offices might be able to accommodate you.

Q: Is it true that most people don't hesitate to use Botox?
A: In the past, before its cosmetic use was FDA approved, people were a little more cautious about Botox and its safety. But today it is commonplace, practically a household word, sometimes even humorously referred to as "vitamin B." As a result, the average patient is really not worried about the treatment and usually has it done.

To Summarize:

- To be safe, get Botox treatments only from a licensed physician with special training and expertise in its use. A board-certified dermatologist, plastic surgeon, ENT facial plastic surgeon, or ophthalmologist with at least several months' experience using Botox on at least a few patients per week is your best choice.

- The two best ways to find a good doctor for Botox treatment are referrals from your regular doctor and recommendations from friends who have already tried Botox and are happy with the results.

- If these methods don't work, some research can usually turn up the names of a few qualified physicians in your area.

- You can obtain information on Botox treatment by calling the doctor's office and talking to a nurse or other staff member.

- A personal consultation in the doctor's office is necessary before you can find out if you are a good candidate for Botox.

- A doctor who is more experienced using Botox is usually preferable to one with less experience.

- If, after the consultation, you and the doctor agree on treatment, you will usually have your first Botox treatment at that time.

- Botox parties are usually not the best way to receive treatment.

- Since FDA approval, Botox treatments are now commonplace and most people do not hesitate to have them.

Chapter 5

What Happens at Your First Visit to the Doctor?

By now, you are pretty well informed about Botox. You have the name of a recommended doctor and you've made an appointment for a consultation—and possibly your first Botox treatment, if all goes well and you decide to proceed. In this chapter, we will talk about how to prepare for your first visit to the doctor, what information to bring with you, what questions the doctor may ask, and what actually happens in the doctor's office.

Q: What should you bring with you on your first visit to the doctor?
A: You will be asked to fill out a medical history form, so you might want to bring notes relating to your health, including any major illnesses or surgery you may have had, any medications you are taking (prescription and

over-the-counter), and any allergies you may have. Also list any herbal products you take on a regular basis.

You might also want to bring a photograph of your mother, especially if you think you look just like her. Some women show me their mother's picture and say, "You know what? I have all my mother's other traits and she has this big groove on her face and she's had it for ten years. So I'm probably going to have it in another ten years, and I'd like to start treating this line now so I can prevent it from getting worse."

Or you could bring a photo of yourself when you were younger so the doctor can see the changes that have taken place in your skin. You might ask the doctor, "Is there any way that these lines I don't like can be improved so I can look the way I did fourteen years ago in this picture?"

These photographs can be very helpful to the physician, but they're not something most people think about when they come in for a visit.

Q: When it comes to the medical forms, can you ask the office to send them in advance so you can fill them out at home?
A: There are some forms that can be mailed or faxed in advance, but most patients prefer to fill them out in the office and it doesn't seem to be a problem. Sometimes when we mail or fax the forms, people forget to bring them in.

You should also realize that for a relatively simple procedure like Botox, you don't need the same kind of detailed information that you need for major surgery.

Q: After the forms are filled out in the office, what happens next?
A: In my practice, the nurse escorts patients in and takes a little more of their medical history after reviewing the forms. When she sees that the patients are scheduled for a Botox consultation, she may ask if they ever had Botox before, if they have friends who have used it, what they know about it, and what they want to accomplish with it.

Q: What does the nurse do with this information?
A: The nurse informs the doctor about what the patients are most interested in regarding Botox treatment so the doctor can focus on this right away. You could say that the nurse is a kind of patient liaison.

Q: What does the doctor do then?
A: The doctor typically comes into the room and asks the same questions all over again! That's not because doctors and nurses don't communicate. This second questioning by the doctor gives patients an opportunity to rethink what they told the nurse and maybe add something or change it. And in fact, this occurs very often.

For instance, they might think of additional questions to ask or more information they want the doctor to provide.

Q: What are some of the questions the doctor asks patients?
A: The doctor will ask the patients, "What are you trying

to accomplish? What is it that we can do for you? What do you want to improve? What questions can we answer?" In that way, we can find out if patients have a clear idea of exactly what they want or if they are uncertain.

If patients are very precise and say, "I'm very unhappy with this particular line," and they point right to it and don't even need a mirror because they know exactly where it is—they see it in the mirror all the time and they hate it—that tells us they are clearly focused on why they want Botox.

Q: When patients are specific like that, what does the doctor do next?

A: At that point the doctor will analyze the skin to determine if there are any contraindications for doing the procedure—that is, any reasons why Botox should not be used. The doctor manipulates the skin to find out if, when it is stretched back, the lines or wrinkles look a little better, or perhaps a lot better.

The doctor will also examine the areas around the lines or wrinkles to try to determine if there are any possibilities that the result would not be as good as expected. Do the eyelids droop? Do the eyebrows go down too far? Is there any asymmetry in the face? Is one eyebrow higher than the other? Is a groove so deep from years of contraction that the patient needs to be informed about the possibility of slow improvement and that collagen injections may also be needed?

When we use Botox, we have to try to balance these things. In fact, Botox can be used for just that purpose, to make each side of the face equal and symmetrical.

Q: What happens if patients are not precise about what they want?
A: Patients who have very vague concepts of what they want may say, "I don't like my face. It looks so old." But they may not be sure that the folds they dislike can benefit from Botox or if they need some other type of treatment.

There's nothing wrong with people being uncertain. That's one reason why they may come in for a consultation—to ask the physician and benefit from his or her expertise.

Q: How do doctors respond in these cases?
A: I usually give people a mirror and point out the differences between the way their faces look now and how they probably looked in the past. I show them the areas where their skin is sagging, where it's thinning, where there are folds, sallowness, cross-hatching, or whatever I find. If there are multiple problems that patients are interested in improving, I point out which ones Botox can address and which ones require a different treatment, such as collagen injections, fat injections, chemical peels, or resurfacing (see chapter 8).

It's important for patients to know that there are additional procedures besides Botox. If they are very interested in doing a microdermabrasion (see chapter 8) that day to smoothen their skin surface, we will not do Botox first. The reason is that the microdermabrasion, by pressing on the skin, could cause the Botox to go to places where we don't want it to go.

So we may say, "After reviewing all your concerns, I think you could benefit most from microdermabrasion and Botox. Since you agree, we definitely need to do the microdermabrasion first, and then when you're finished, we can inject the Botox." This is actually a very common scenario.

Q: Is it always effective for the doctor to suggest various treatments to patients?
A: No, not always. Sometimes patients will tell me, "I have this line and I've wanted to come in for some time to have Botox. I have a wedding tonight, or I have to give a lecture, or I have a television appearance, and I really want to look my best." Unfortunately, I have to inform them that it is never a good idea to have Botox the same day as an important event.

Q: Why not?
A: Botox doesn't work that quickly. It puts you at risk for little bumps in the areas that are injected and you most likely will not look your best the same night after your injections. And it also takes several days to reach its full effect. Lines will not disappear completely in a few hours and there is also a very slight chance of temporary bruising.

Q: What is the best schedule?
A: With Botox, you should give yourself at least twenty-four to forty-eight hours before any important event to allow your skin to recover. But you should also remember that it can take one to two weeks for the full effects of Botox to appear, so it's best to have the shots at least two weeks before an important event.

Q: Are there other reasons why physicians would decide not to use Botox on the first visit?

A: If patients are taking one of the nonsteroidal medications, like Motrin or Advil, perhaps for back pain, and they definitely do not want any bruising, it is better for them to come back after not using these medications for a few days. Otherwise, there will be a much higher risk of bruising.

Q: Are there other substances you should avoid prior to Botox treatment?

A: If you absolutely want to avoid any chance of bruising, you should avoid alcohol for at least twenty-four hours, and aspirin and vitamin E for about two weeks. These substances can increase the risk of bruising because they are all blood thinners.

Q: What about blood-thinning medications, such as Coumadin and Plavix?

A: In cases like these, physicians have to contact the prescribing doctor and discuss the situation. You would not want to put someone at risk by taking them off a needed medication so they can have a cosmetic procedure and avoid bruising. And of course, *no patient should ever stop taking a medication without first consulting the prescribing physician.*

Q: Do any other over-the-counter products have this same blood-thinning effect?

A: There are some holistic herbs that can increase the

risk of bruising, such as ginger, *Gingko biloba*, garlic, and ginseng—in supplement form. To avoid bruising, you should not take any of these herbal supplements for about two weeks prior to your Botox treatment.

Q: What are some of the reasons that might make you decide patients are not good Botox candidates?
A: If they have a very deep groove, and when we stretch the skin, that deep line does not come up, there is a high chance that patients will not be happy with the result. If they point to their lower face, to the areas of the smile folds, or if they point to the cross marks on their cheeks, neither of which is going to respond to Botox, then of course they are not candidates.

Or, if they want the lines on their foreheads treated, but they already have a very low forehead and their eyelids risk obstructing their vision if they come down, then you really can't use Botox on those lines.

Q: When you pull the facial skin in the office before the Botox treatment, can patients see exactly how they will look after the treatment is fully effective?
A: Not really. Because the results are usually much better than that. Pulling the skin is just a clue that the area is going to get better, but we can't simulate the result precisely. It takes time for the Botox to achieve its full effect. As time goes on after treatment, the skin gets more and more smooth and the wrinkling diminishes. You just have to wait and see how good the results are when the full effect is finally attained.

Q: Do before-and-after pictures of other patients give a good idea of the results?
A: Yes, they give a good general idea. But again, every individual is different, so you can't know exactly what your results with Botox will be until you try it.

Q: If you decide that the patients are good candidates, they understand the details of Botox treatment and they want to try it, do you inject them following this consultation period?
A: Yes. That's the way it happens with most of my patients.

To Summarize:

- For your first visit to the doctor, bring information on your medical history and consider bringing a photograph of a parent or close relative who looks like you, or a photograph of a younger you if you think this is relevant to your concerns about your skin.

- Be ready to tell the nurse and the doctor why you are there, what areas of your face bother you, and what you hope to achieve with Botox.

- Be prepared with any questions you want to ask the doctor.

- Remember that Botox can't treat every skin problem and the doctor may recommend other treatments for some of your concerns.

• You should never have Botox on the same day you want to look good. Botox can take one to two weeks or more before you can see its full effect. In addition, the red bumps that sometimes form on the injection sites can take many hours to disappear. Give yourself at least two full days before an important event.

• Avoid alcohol for one day and nonsteroidal medications like Motrin and Advil for a few days before using Botox. Avoid aspirin, vitamin E, and the herbal supplements gingko, ginger, garlic, and ginseng for two weeks. All of these can cause bruising because of their blood-thinning effects. You or the doctor's office should check with your physician about any prescription blood-thinning medication you may be taking, but never stop taking it on your own before going for a Botox consultation.

Chapter 6

What Happens During Your First Botox Treatment?

You've passed your examination with flying colors. You feel comfortable with the doctor you've selected, and both of you agree that Botox is a good treatment for the lines or wrinkles that are bothering you. You feel confident that this is exactly what you want, and you decide to go ahead and have your first Botox treatment right then and there.

This chapter will describe the actual Botox treatment—how the doctor and nurse prepare you for the injections, how they are given, what the procedure feels like, how long it takes, the length of the recovery period, and what you should and should not do following treatment.

Q: How is the face prepared in the doctor's office before Botox treatment?
A: My patients are in a sitting position, just slightly reclined, and their skin is cleaned with alcohol. Soothing

music is playing in the background. The correct lighting is used to show the lines—not so bright as to hurt the eyes, but just enough to create the right shadows to highlight the creases. We often put a numbing cream on the face, a topical anesthetic, and have the patients wait about thirty minutes for it to take effect.

Is this cream necessary? Not really. There are some patients who find that the Botox injections don't hurt them at all and they can have the treatment without an anesthetic cream. Other people are in a hurry and don't have the time to wait for the cream to take effect. So the cream is just an added benefit for those patients who want it.

Q: How long do the effects of the numbing cream last? Does the face feel uncomfortable during this time?
A: The effects last for one or more hours. Some people say the area feels a little heavy, slightly strange or uncomfortable, but this does not seem to bother people.

Q: Do people have pain when they are injected with Botox, either with or without the numbing cream?
A: Some people do have a little pain. After all, we are putting a needle through the skin and into the muscle. It's a very fine needle and it's not very long. You will feel a little bit of a sting when the needle goes in.

Some people describe it as similar to an insect bite, while others feel a very slight burning sensation. But many people say they don't feel anything or may remark, "That's not bad at all." For the vast majority, Botox injections are very tolerable and the treatment does not take long.

Q: Is it necessary to mark the spots on the face that will be injected?
A: No. Some doctors may do this, but the majority do not. In the first place, surgical markers leave visible spots on the face and most people do not want any downtime. They don't want any marks on their faces and they don't want to have to explain to anyone that they have had a cosmetic procedure.

In the second place, the marks do not come off easily, and we don't want patients rubbing their skin and possibly spreading the Botox to places where it should not go.

If doctors can put a marker in the place that's going to be injected, they can also put the needle in the same spot and just inject. You only need to know where the muscles are and then inject them.

Q: Are there special ways to determine the location of the exact spot to inject?
A: The physician needs to know the anatomy of the face. I also find that if patients move and grimace, it's easier to find the right spot because I can see the specific details of their individual anatomies. Not everyone is exactly the same.

Q: What do you ask them to do?
A: I have the patients grimace so I can see their lines—say, between their brows. I show them with my face what I want them to do—push the eyebrows together in what I call a "scrunch." Next I look for the "belly" (the fleshy part that contracts) of the muscle to stick out; then I have them scrunch again and use my fingers to feel the spot.

By doing this, I can get an idea of the thickness of their muscle and its midpoint, which is where I am going to inject. In most patients, there are standard spots. But for a lot of areas on the forehead, especially between the eyebrows, it's helpful for me to see exactly where those bellies are jutting up.

There are three muscle groups that control the wrinkling between the eyebrows and it's important to find and inject all three of those muscles, especially in men and women who have what are called hypertrophic (or enlarged) muscles. People with these types of muscles often need more units of Botox.

Q: How many injections of Botox are needed for the three most common procedures?
A: For the glabellar area between the eyebrows, we generally use five to seven; for the crow's-feet around the eyes, it's usually two or three per side; and for the lines in the forehead, it can be anywhere from eight to fifteen or more injections.

Q: How many units of Botox do those represent?
A: Between the brows, it is from twenty-five to thirty-five units; for the crow's-feet, six to fifteen units per side or twelve to thirty total units; and for the forehead, eighteen to fifty units or more. In some cases, of course, more units and more injections are required.

Q: How does the skin react when the Botox injections are given?

A: Usually, there is a small amount of swelling. After all, fluid is going in and it has to go somewhere. So the skin forms a little red bump where the needle comes out, and typically, that's all there is. This swelling usually goes down after a few hours.

Q: What about bleeding?
A: Occasionally there is a small amount of blood, but it typically stops when we apply just a little pressure for about twenty to thirty seconds at most.

Q: Do people ever have any other reactions to Botox injections? Do they ever feel dizzy or ill during treatment?
A: That hasn't happened in my office yet. There are patients who faint at the sight of a needle, but they usually don't come in for elective treatments requiring injections, such as Botox.

Q: What happens after the Botox injections? How long do patients have to remain in the office?
A: We typically give our patients a small ice compress for about a minute to help minimize the little red bumps where the needle went in. We don't want to overice though, so after about a minute we have the patients stand up, walk out, and perhaps go to the bathroom and put on a little makeup or fix their hair if they want to.

Q: How long does the actual treatment last?
A: Without the time for the numbing cream to take effect,

the actual treatment, on average, lasts from two to twenty minutes. The exact time depends on which sites and how many areas are being injected, as well as a patient's preferences for taking breaks or discussing each area before it is treated.

Q: Is it all right to apply makeup right after treatment?
A: Usually that's fine, unless there is a little bleeding area. Then patients should avoid putting makeup around that little dot until it is completely dry.

Q: What happens next?
A: If it's their first Botox treatment, I always ask patients to come in again in two to four weeks so I can evaluate their results. In fact, there are some patients who only realize a full effect after one month. But after the second treatment, they don't have to come in between treatments unless they don't see the same good results they had with their first session.

Of course, if patients have any questions, they are encouraged to call and discuss their concerns at any time.

Q: Are there any precautions or rules patients have to follow after Botox treatment?
A: There are some things we ask patients to do in the first four hours following treatment. We tell them not to bend over, lie down, or dramatically change their position because that could move the Botox around. For the same reason, they should not have any facials or massages on

the area that has been injected. You don't want to do any kind of massage technique or manipulation to the area that has been treated for fear of spreading the Botox, making it affect muscles that we don't want affected, such as causing the eyelid muscles to droop.

Patients should not go to a facialist, at whose office their pores might be expressed using heat on the skin. And when they wash their face that night, they should be very gentle, never rough.

They should not cook over a hot stove for a few hours after Botox because the heat could weaken its effect. We also recommend that they do not wear tight-collared tops that have to be pulled over the head because such a garment can squeeze the skin as the top comes off and perhaps manipulate the Botox into different locations where we do not want it to spread.

We also ask them to do a little facial exercise for the first hour after treatment. By scrunching their muscles, patients can purposely move the particular muscles that they want to be eventually inhibited by the Botox. It is wise for patients to actively move these muscles—not with their fingers, but using the actual muscle—for the first hour after treatment so those muscles can incorporate the Botox.

Q: Do some people come in for Botox on their lunch hours and then go back to work?
A: Some people do.

Q: So nobody at work will notice anything when they get back to the office?

A: There are very slight pink to red dots or bumps. Because of this, some patients prefer to come for treatment in the late afternoon and not return to work. In the case of many patients, it is impossible to tell that they've just had a Botox treatment. So it's an individual decision based on how you feel and how you look immediately after treatment.

To Summarize:

• Botox injections are not normally painful, but you can have a numbing cream applied if you so choose.

• When you are injected with Botox, you may feel a slight sting or burning sensation, but many people don't feel anything.

• The doctor can locate the correct spots for injection by having you make certain facial expressions, such as grimacing.

• Depending on what area is treated, you may need from four to fifteen or more injections per area.

• After each injection, there is usually a small bump or swelling, which normally goes away in a few hours. There is very little bleeding, if any.

• A typical treatment takes from two to twenty minutes per area. If numbing cream is used, it takes about thirty minutes to take effect prior to the actual treatment.

- Patients return for follow-up visits two to four weeks after the first treatment to check the results.

- If the first treatment succeeds, the average person returns for further Botox treatments every three to four months.

- Do not bend over, have facial massages, manipulate the treated area, cook over a hot stove, or pull a tight-collared top over your head for the first four hours after Botox treatment.

- Most people prefer to have Botox treatments after work so they can go home while their swelling gradually goes down.

- Several times in the first hours after Botox, you should actively contract your muscles in the way your doctor shows you so the Botox will be drawn into the neuromuscular junction and can be more effective.

Below is a sample consent form for cosmetic Botox treatment, similar to one you may be asked to sign before receiving your first treatment:

CONSENT TO BOTOX TREATMENT FOR FACIAL WRINKLES

Rationale: I am aware that when small amounts of purified botulinum toxin ("Botox") are injected into a muscle, they cause weakness or paralysis of that muscle. This may appear in three to four days, but may take up to one month to show full effect. Botox usually lasts four months, but the length of time can be shorter or longer.

Some lines on the face are due to contraction of a small muscle beneath the skin. Injecting Botox into these muscles will paralyze them, causing improvement or disappearance of frown lines.

FDA Approval: Botox is approved by the Food and Drug Administration for use in neuromuscular disorders, eye muscle problems, and frown lines between the eyebrows. Although it is legal for my physician to use Botox for improving other facial lines, the FDA has not yet approved Botox for treating crow's-feet lines, forehead lines, or other muscle-related lines on the face and neck.

Results and Postoperative Care:

1. I understand that I will not be able to frown while the injection is effective, but that this will reverse itself after a period of months, at which time retreatment is appropriate.

2. I understand that I must stay in an erect position and that I must not manipulate the area of the injection for the four-hour postinjection period.

3. For four hours after Botox treatment, I will not exercise, bend over, massage the areas of treatment, take a long walk, wash or color my hair, wear a cap or a hat, apply or remove makeup, pull clothing off over my head, go shopping for

shoes (which may require bending over), or cook over a hot stove.

Risks and Complications: Botox treatment of frown lines can cause a minor temporary droop of one eyelid in approximately 2 percent of injections. This usually lasts two to three weeks. Occasional numbness of the forehead lasting two to three weeks, bruising, and transient headaches have also occurred.

In a very small number of individuals, Botox injections do not work as satisfactorily or for as long as usual.

Contraindicated conditions: I am not aware that I am pregnant, breast-feeding, or have any neurologic disease.

Chapter 7

What Results Will You Get and How Can You Maintain Them?

You've done it! You've made your decision, found a good doctor, had your consultation and undergone your first Botox treatment. It didn't take long and it didn't even hurt. You followed your doctor's recommendations and the first four hours have gone by. What should you expect now?

This chapter will tell you what results you can anticipate from your Botox treatment. We will go into detail about the possible side effects that you might experience, discuss how Botox can affect facial expressions, and tell you what to do if you are not happy with your results or if you don't get any results at all.

Q: After the first four hours following Botox treatment, are there any special things patients should do?
A: You should still be gentle washing your face. After

four hours, the little bumps usually have gone down, but
it's still wise to take precautions. Other than that, people
can just resume their normal routines.

**Q: How long does it take to see visible results after
the first Botox treatment?**
A: It really takes anywhere from several days to up to
two weeks, and on rare occasions even longer—perhaps
a month or so—to see the full effects of that first treatment.

**Q: Are the results from the first treatment different
from those of subsequent treatments?**
A: It's important to know that there can be better results
with continued Botox treatments. If you have a second
treatment just as the first one is starting to wear off, but
not much longer, those improved creases in the skin will
not have the chance to re-create themselves, and they will
actually improve with subsequent treatments.

But if you wait and allow the skin a chance to form
those creases again, then the line re-forms much more
readily. So as soon as you begin to be able to move those
muscles again, you should make an appointment for another Botox treatment.

**Q: Why does it take so much time to see results? Ex-
actly what is the Botox doing in the muscles that creates the need to wait for lines and wrinkles to
disappear?**
A: The nerve has a certain supply of acetylcholine, the

chemical messenger that is used to create communication between the nerve and the muscle. You have to wait for this chemical to be used up.

Botox is a competitive inhibitor. That means it blocks newer chemical messengers from being received by the receptors. So the reason you have to wait is for some of the neural chemical messengers to be used up. Botox actually attaches to the receptors so they can be blocked, and at a certain point the muscle won't be able to function.

Q: What is the result that the physician wishes to achieve with Botox?
A: Botox prevents the muscle from moving, so the lines and wrinkles can't form from the movement of those muscles, and as a consequence, the skin becomes smoother.

For instance, if we prevent the muscles in our forehead from raising the forehead up, or prevent the muscles controlling our eyebrows from making them come together, or prevent the muscles that cause us to squint from being able to do that, we will prevent all these actions and then those lines will diminish.

Q: How do the lines diminish?
A: They diminish in two ways. The first is the immediate effect of taking the deeper furrow or fold and having it smooth out because the muscle is not actively contracting it.

At the same time, on the surface of that furrow is a separate superficial crease, and that crease has been formed by repetitive motions of the muscle and the skin folding on itself. So the deeper folds will improve more readily as the Botox minimizes the muscle movement. But the little crease that's been formed over a long period is going to take a long time to go away, because you have to wait for the collagen in the dermis to re-form itself, to be produced more, and to create a more orderly arrangement so the skin doesn't form that little crease.

Q: What are some of the possible side effects of Botox treatment?
A: Virtually everyone has lightly swollen pinkish bumps where the injections went in for a couple of hours. It's important to know that because makeup won't hide a slight elevation of the skin, you should not have Botox two hours before you have a big dinner date. But if you have Botox the day before, it's usually no problem.

Q: Aside from that, what is the most common side effect?
A: Although many people with chronic headaches or migraines often get relief from Botox, a small percent of patients get headaches following treatment, for the first evening. This is more typical when we work on the lines of the forehead than when we put Botox on the area between the eyebrows or around the eyes.

Headaches might also be dependent on the method of injection. If the Botox is injected very deeply, down to the bone, there may be a much greater chance of headaches developing.

One study reported five patients whose post-Botox headaches lasted up to five days, but again, this is very unusual. All these patients had Botox treatments on their foreheads.

Q: What are the other side-effect possibilities?
A: There can be a lowering of the eyelids after the Botox takes effect. And very rarely, there can be temporary double vision. Some other side effects recorded in studies include flulike symptoms, back pain, respiratory problems such as bronchitis or sinusitis, nausea, dizziness, and tightness or irritation of the skin. These reported side effects occurred in a very small number of people, under 3 percent of test subjects in most studies, and were not greater in number than the side effects in patients who were tested with a placebo (a saline solution without Botox). The only significant side effect was headache, affecting about 13 percent of the test subjects.

There is another risk when injecting Botox around the eyes. Paralyzing the muscles here, as is done when Botox is used medically to treat blepharospasm, can lead to corneal exposure because people may not be able to blink their eyelids as often as they should to protect the eye.

There is also a risk in injecting Botox around the mouth, which is why it is not normally used in that area. With muscles weakened, side effects like drooling or the inability to properly enunciate words can result.

Finally, Allergan, the manufacturer of Botox, lists some of the very rare adverse reactions as including rare spontaneous reports of death, sometimes associated with dysphagia (swallowing problems), pneumonia, cardiac arrhythmia, and myocardial infarction. Some of the people who experienced these rare reactions had preexisting diseases, and no direct connection with the use of Botox has

been established. Probability suggests that these occur-
rences were coincidences and would have occurred even
if Botox was not given.

All these reactions, by the way, were associated with
the use of medical Botox. I am not aware of any such
reactions with cosmetic Botox, which, as we know, is
given in a much lower dose. You should also know that
an antidote is available for severe reactions to Botox.

Q: In your practice, have you seen many side effects?
A: Very rarely. I had one patient who developed a fever
of 101 degrees within an hour of treatment but was fine
in a matter of hours. I have no idea if this was related to
the Botox, but almost all of my patients experience no
unpleasant or troublesome side effects.

Q: What about bruising?
A: If you avoid the substances we've mentioned that can
create a greater likelihood of bruising, the chances are
minimal when the procedure goes smoothly. There's always a slight chance of bruising anytime you inject anything, but the area that is most prone to bruising is the
area around the eyes when we treat the crow's-feet. Because the skin in this area is thin, it is far more likely to
bruise than the thicker skin on the forehead or between
the brows.

**Q: Can you cover up the marks of bruising with
makeup?**
A: Sometimes you can, but on other occasions, the bruis-

ing is such that it is not easily covered by most makeup. In those cases, you can use a special cream or foundation, such as Dermablend or Covermark.

Bruising is partly dependent on the physician's technique, but not completely. Sometimes patients will bruise and there's not a lot you can do about it—just cover it up and wait until it heals.

Q: You mentioned a possible droopy eyelid after Botox. What causes that?
A: When treating the forehead, there is about a 2 percent chance of one of the eyelids lowering by a thirty-second or a sixteenth of an inch. This lowering eyelid does not tend to cover the pupil of the eye completely, but it can encroach on the top edge of the pupil. If it does, when people are walking straight ahead, they may not, for example, be able to see that cabinet in the kitchen that is hanging down and could walk into it. But even when this eyelid droop occurs, it is temporary and is usually gone within three weeks. Iopidine, an eyedrop medication, may lift the eyelid a millimeter or so and can help in the meantime, but sometimes the droop is too great and the eyedrops are not really effective.

Q: What are some of the side effects you have seen?
A: One woman said her forehead came down a little bit, but it was not obstructing her vision and she had no problem with it. Another woman had Botox that did not adequately affect the side of her forehead and one eyebrow was still able to be elevated, giving her what we sometimes call "the Jack Nicholson effect." By adding a little

Botox to that side, the problem was solved and her brows were equalized.

Q: After your first Botox treatment, can your face change very dramatically or are the changes more subtle? Will you be able to make the same facial expressions as before or will you find you can't because the muscles are paralyzed?
A: We don't really use much Botox in the lower two-thirds of the face, as a rule. There are exceptions and there are some individual reasons why we might use it in small amounts in a focal area, but you should be able to smile, enunciate, purse your lips, and make most of the facial expressions you have made in the past.

Even when we treat the forehead, there is still some subtle movement in most of my patients. So yes, you may not be able to frown or scowl the way you used to, but you had Botox treatment to purposely inhibit your ability to make those expressions. Only in this way can the lines and wrinkles fade.

Typically, the faces of Botox patients do not change dramatically if the drug is administered according to the recommendations. Patients do not look like they have stone faces. They still have a natural appearance, but their skin looks younger, smoother, and more even.

But if actors came to me for Botox before trying out for a part, I would make certain they realize that if they have to make a very angry expression or look quizzical or raise their eyebrows, they may not be able to do so after Botox. The same is true for a television newscaster or anyone who needs to make a variety of facial expressions for a specific purpose.

Q: But we hear that almost everyone in the media has had cosmetic treatments, including Botox. Isn't that true?
A: I'm not sure if it's true or not. You often can't tell just by looking at people. There is a way of being conservative with Botox, using just enough and in just the right places so there is still sufficient muscle movement to be facially expressive. When this is done, people often look quite natural and almost the same as before.

But some people aren't happy with a very small amount and may want greater changes. In such cases, patients who have had very little Botox may come back another time for more treatment. This method is much better than giving patients too much initially and taking the risk of creating an artificial look.

Q: When your patients come back after their first Botox treatment, do they let you know what their friends and family have said? Do they normally tell people they have had Botox or try to keep it a secret?
A: Many times other people will notice a difference and ask the patients if they have been away on vacation because they look so well rested. Or they may say, "You look so good. What's going on in your life that has changed?" Or, "Did you get a new hairstyle?" and so on, because the individual looks more upbeat and serene.

As to whether Botox patients tell other people about the procedure, I'd estimate that about half do and half don't. But in almost every case, the changes are subtle rather than dramatic, so it's hard for other people to figure out exactly what has changed.

Q: So their friends think they are just better rested or happier?
A: Yes, because most of us are not so observant that we remember every line in another person's face. We don't say, "Oh, Jane had two hills and a valley between her eyebrows. What happened to them?"

Instead, Jane's acquaintances might remember that for whatever reason, Jane never seemed to be in a good mood for the past several years (because she was always frowning without realizing it and had deep creases between her brows). Now, all of a sudden, they observe that she seems more relaxed and happy.

Q: And what do the patients say about how they feel?
A: Very often they say they have more confidence in themselves. Nothing else has changed, but the grimace they kept making or the lines they hated are not there anymore.

They remark that they feel more relaxed in social situations and have a greater feeling of self-esteem.

Q: What should patients do if they are not happy with their results? What if they don't look the way they wanted to or the way they expected to after the full effect has taken place?
A: These patients should always go back to their doctor. You must return to the original doctor first in order to find out what's going on. If you go to another doctor, that second doctor is handicapped because he or she doesn't know where the Botox was delivered, how many units were used, what dilution was given, and so on.

Many things can be analyzed and repaired. So you have to discuss your results with the doctor who treated you and then find out if your results can be improved.

Q: How can that be done?
A: If it's a lack of completion—that is, if there are other areas that need treatment—then those areas can be injected. If you need a larger dose, we can inject additional Botox.

So it's important to go back to the same doctor and explain what is bothering you, and the chances are, it can be corrected. But keep in mind that any units of Botox in subsequent treatments may cost you more.

Q: Is it possible to have Botox treatment and to have no results at all?
A: Yes, that can happen. There are a number of reasons why, but the patient should return to the doctor and have an assessment. Sometimes the first treatment doesn't work, but the second one will have the desired results. It requires an individual diagnosis.

Q: How do people know when they need another treatment? Is it when they feel their muscles moving again?
A: That's right. Some people can feel it and other people look in the mirror periodically, and when they see that they can make grimaces again, for instance, then they know the muscle is contracting again and they need more Botox.

Q: Is there a typical schedule for people to return for more Botox treatments?
A: Three to four months is the average, especially in the beginning, but some people's effects last for five or six months. And as time goes on and treatments continue, they can last for an even longer time. So after several years of treatments, the Botox could last for six or seven or possibly even eight months.

Some patients have claimed that for them, Botox lasts for a full year, but I have not seen this in my office. In my experience, the range is three to five months and, very rarely, six months.

Q: If you get Botox treatments over a long period of time, say five years or more, your body is aging at the same time. So after five years, will you still be getting the same effect when you are injected?
A: We think you will. There is no reason to think that the Botox wouldn't work just as well.

Q: So your face will look just as young five years down the road?
A: Well, there are other factors at issue besides chronological aging, and those factors are not addressed by Botox. They include sun exposure, lack of sleep, smoking, and things like that. But if everything else remains equal and you take good care of yourself, that nice, smooth skin can be maintained if you keep up your Botox treatment schedule.

Q: Remind us of what problems can occur if someone comes in for Botox too often or goes to more than one doctor to get extra Botox?

A: Overexposure to Botox can cause the body to produce antibodies and then the Botox may no longer be effective. We have no evidence that excessive use can cause the body to develop an allergy to Botox, but it is a possibility. It's much wiser to stick to your doctor's recommended schedule for your treatments.

Q: So most people can expect to continue using Botox for the rest of their lives if they want to, as long as they do so on the correct schedule and follow their physician's recommendations?

A: That's right. So far, we have no information to indicate anything to the contrary.

To Summarize:

* It can take from several days to two weeks or more to see the visible results of Botox.

* Treatments after the first one can yield better results.

* You should have your next Botox treatment just as the first one is wearing off and you are able to move your facial muscles again. Waiting longer will allow unwanted lines to form again and possibly deepen.

- Botox has few side effects. Most people have lightly swollen pinkish bumps on the injection sites, which last a few hours, and some may have temporary bruising. A small number get headaches, especially with forehead treatment, and a few may have droopy eyelids. There are other possible side effects, but they affect less than 3 percent of patients.

- When used properly, the effects of Botox are subtle and you will still be able to be facially expressive, but not in an extreme way that causes lines and creases to form.

- After Botox, most people look happier, more serene, and better rested. Friends may comment on this, even though they aren't aware of the treatment. About half of Botox patients tell others and half do not.

- Botox patients frequently report feeling more self-confident and relaxed in social situations.

- If you aren't happy with your results or don't get any results at all (a rarity), return to the same doctor and ask that a solution be worked out.

- With continued treatments over about five years, many people's results last six months or more.

- It appears to be safe to use Botox for a lifetime.

Chapter 8

What Other Cosmetic Medical Procedures Can Erase the Signs of Aging?

Although Botox is an amazing drug that has worked wonders for millions of people who want to reverse the signs of aging on their faces, it is not the only effective treatment. Patients have quite a few options to choose from, and with the guidance of an experienced physician, they can select the best treatment for whatever problems are bothering them.

In this chapter, we will look at a few of the more popular treatments. Some can be used for areas where Botox is not effective, others can be used in combination with Botox, and still others may be selected as alternatives to Botox.

Q: Are there any other products similar to Botox?

A: There is a product called Myobloc, which is derived from botulinum toxin B. It is made by Elan Pharmaceu-

ticals, an Irish company, and has been approved by the
FDA to treat cervical dystonia, the disorder that causes
neck muscles to contract involuntarily. It has also been
used off-label to treat facial lines and wrinkles. Myobloc
takes effect more quickly than Botox, sometimes in
twenty-four hours, but, according to several doctors, the
effects don't seem to last as long at the current dosages.

We mentioned the possibility of people forming antibodies to Botox if they use it for many years, although
this occurs in only about 5 percent of Botox patients. If
this happens, these people could then use Myobloc because the antibodies would not attack the B type of the
toxin that is in Myobloc, only the A type that is in Botox.

Another similar product is Dysport, a drug made by
Ipsen Ltd., a British company. It is composed of *Clostridium botulinum* toxin A–hemagglutinin complex, and
also contains albumin and lactose. It is used for treatments
of certain medical disorders, including blepharospasm and
pediatric cerebral palsy.

**Q: Other than these, what are the treatment options
that patients can choose instead of Botox? And if Botox is such a great drug, why would anybody want to
use them?**
A: There are other products available that some people
may use instead of Botox. To understand the situation
better, we should look at three main areas: (1) what was
available before Botox existed; (2) what products can be
used for wrinkles that don't respond to Botox; and (3)
what products can be used to enhance the results we get
with Botox and improve areas that have been damaged by
the sun.

Q: What treatments were used for wrinkles before Botox was available?

A: At that time the areas of fine lines around the eyes, the deep creases between the eyebrows, and the forehead creases—all the areas now treated by Botox—were treated with collagen injections. And collagen injections can help these areas, there is no doubt about it.

Q: What kind of collagen is used?

A: As we already mentioned, collagen is a protein substance in the dermis layer of the skin as well as in our tendons, bones, and cartilage. It is largely responsible for the skin's integrity, and when it is damaged or lost over time, it results in the skin wrinkling and sagging.

But the collagen that we inject for cosmetic purposes is pure bovine collagen. It comes from cows that are kept in a closed herd so they cannot be infected by mad cow disease or other disorders. The cows are constantly tested to be certain they are healthy, and the collagen is produced by a sterile process.

Q: How is this collagen used?

A: Some people—about 3 percent of the population—are allergic to bovine collagen. So first, the patient has to have two skin tests to make certain that there is no collagen allergy. These tests are separated by a few weeks. If both skin tests indicate no allergy, the risk of a reaction goes down to 1.5 percent.

Q: What happens if someone has an allergic reaction?

A: It is not life-threatening. There's a red bump that appears where the collagen was injected. It can form many days after the injection and can last as long as nine months or more.

Q: How does the collagen work in the skin?
A: Collagen is a filler. If we have a wrinkle and put something underneath it to raise up the skin, this filler will smooth out the wrinkle. There are many different types of fillers, but collagen is the most popular.

The collagen we inject is temporary, and like Botox, it has to be periodically reinjected to maintain the effect of plumping up the wrinkles. Collagen injections last about four months on average, and rarely more than six months. When collagen is injected into an area that moves a lot, like the lips, it may only last for a month.

Q: How long does it take for collagen to take full effect?
A: Most people are fine by the next day.

Q: What are some of the other fillers that have been used?
A: Medical-grade silicone has been used in the past, with physicians using a microdroplet technique, where just enough is put into the skin to correct the problem. But silicone is rarely used today, although doctors can use a new form for off-label applications, since it is FDA approved for use by ophthalmologists to inject into the eye for certain medical conditions.

Q: Why isn't silicone used so often anymore?
A: Unlike collagen, which is temporary, silicone is permanent. There have been concerns about its possible adverse effect on the immune system, although there is no scientific proof that it is dangerous in that way.

But silicone can also form "silicone granulomas," which are small inflamed nodules under the skin. We are not certain why they form, but there could be an adulterant in the silicone, or the silicone could create antibodies that provoke an autoimmune response.

Q: Other than collagen, what fillers are now in use?
A: New fillers are currently being developed. There are some that have been used in Europe for some time and may soon be approved by the FDA for use in this country. They include Hylaform and Hylaform Plus, which can be used on facial lines, wrinkles, and lips. This product is a modified form of hyaluronic acid, a naturally occurring substance in the human skin and body, which is the actual ground substance or fluid component of the dermis. It is absorbed into the body, so treatments have to be repeated once or twice a year after the initial treatment.

The dermis, the infrastructure of the skin, is composed of collagen (a protein network), which is lying in a sort of shock-absorber protective viscous gel-like fluid. So Hylaform is made from a substance that we actually produce in our own bodies.

Other similar products, Restylane and Perlane, are made from recombinant DNA in the laboratory by a Swedish company. They are really the same product, but Perlane comes in a larger dosage. They are long-lasting gels made from a substance similar to the body's hyaluronic acid, which is extracted from roosters' combs. These products are injected into the skin with a very thin needle, much like collagen, to plump up or raise the skin to fill in wrinkles and lines (including smile folds), enhance lips, and reshape facial contours. Again, the injected substance dissolves over time and the treatment has to be repeated, usually about six months after the first treatment. Because these products use a substance close to one found in our bodies, allergic reactions are much less likely than with collagen, which is derived from animals. But, like collagen, they can also cause bruising, redness, and swelling.

Q: Do these products give you better effects than Botox?
A: On the forehead, fillers don't give you as smooth an effect as when the muscle is relaxed with Botox. When we inject Botox and it takes effect after a few weeks, the lines almost totally disappear.

But with these collagen products, the lines are less apparent, but they do not disappear. They can also be bumpy sometimes because you are putting something under the skin that is not the exact same texture as your normal skin. So when you run your finger over the area with the filler, you feel little lumps and bumps.

This is especially evident in the thin skin around the eyes where the crow's-feet are located. Sometimes you can even see these little lumps.

Q: Now that physicians have Botox, will they stop using collagen?
A: Collagen is not commonly used on the forehead or

crow's-feet anymore. But it is still being used in the glabellar area between the eyebrows. So people who have
really deep folds between their eyebrows, even when they
are relaxed and at rest, can benefit.

We can use what is called a "sandwich treatment,"
combining Botox and collagen, one above and the other
below. But in other areas, such as the smile folds around
the mouth, we can't use Botox.

Q: Why not?
A: Botox in that area can weaken the muscle and the
crease will flatten a little bit; it can also change the shape
of the face when you smile. As you may recall, it can
even cause drooling and an inability to enunciate words
correctly when injected into muscles of the lips.

Q: Can collagen be used for creases in the neck?
A: Yes, you can use it, but again, little lumps sometimes
form, and because of this, you can see the line somewhat.
Botox, on the other hand, will smoothen the line and make
everything look more natural.

**Q: What was done for the forehead lines before Bo-
tox?**
A: Many people had a surgical brow-lift, where a surgeon
goes in and cuts some muscles. If there is a lot of excess
skin, some of that skin can also be cut out and sewn back
together so it will be tighter. But not everyone wants to
have facial surgery, and Botox has given people another
option.

**Q: After Botox injections, how do you decide what
other treatments you want to use?**
A: Sometimes after patients have Botox treatments on the
forehead, for example, they no longer focus on that area.
They may start to look at other areas and find wrinkles
they don't like.

There might be deep smile folds or wrinkles on the
upper lip, areas where we do not use Botox. So then we
can start talking about different treatments. But first we
have to determine what kinds of lines we are going to
treat.

Q: What about smile folds?
A: If you have very minimal smile folds, then collagen
can be a good choice. If the smile folds are moderate,
then you can still use collagen, but it can become expensive because you have to use more. But for deep folds,
the cost can become prohibitive. You may need four syringes of collagen, which can cost over $1,200 and may
last only a few months.

**Q: So what can you do for the person with deep smile
folds?**
A: One option is fat injections. The fat is taken from the
patient and is not shared among patients. Very often, it is
used for people who have had collagen injections for
many years and want something that will be more cost-
effective.

Injecting fat is actually a graft, and there is a chance
that the fat cells will now live in a new environment. We
take the fat from the buttock area, the belly area, or the

thigh area, prepare it in the laboratory, and then inject it in the area where it is needed.

So on the smile folds, for example, a very tiny nick is made in the skin and a very small catheter is introduced. Then we insert the fat. We layer it in the deep and middle layers, but we are not injecting it superficially. By that I mean that we are not putting it into the epidermis or the superficial dermis; we are injecting it into the deeper dermis and the fatty layer.

So using fat in this way is not the same as injecting collagen, which is injected more superficially. That's why someone who has really deep smile folds, for example, and has been using lots of collagen, is a good candidate for fat. The fat injection is a living graft, and after the first transfer, we may get a 10 percent take, meaning that 10 percent of the fat we inject remains there and lives in its new environment.

The next time we inject the fat, there is an even better chance that more will take. There's now better circulation, new blood vessels have grown in the area, and there is a better host for the new fat to become a permanent part of your body. And so on with each treatment, until we attain the full effect the patient is looking for.

Q: How often can fat be injected?
A: It varies. Some doctors inject fat every month, and others, such as myself, prefer to inject it at intervals of several months. The treatments might be six or even nine months apart, because I think that this type of treatment has to be modified based on the patient's individual results.

So if a patient comes back after a first injection of fat,

and a good amount of the fat has taken and the result looks nice, there is no reason to rush. Give it more time and let whatever portion of the injected fat that is going to take get settled in and then add more when the fat that is not going to take has left the body.

Q: Are fat injections painful?
A: The procedure involves a local anesthetic; sedation is not needed. Patients experience an occasional twinge of discomfort as the fat goes in.

When we are taking the fat out of the body for preparation, we also use a local anesthetic.

Q: Does the fat get injected back in right away?
A: Some physicians do that, but I prefer to centrifuge it, which helps separate out the unwanted fluids, including the anesthetic. In that way, I know that when I put the fat back into the body, it is in a similar state to the one it was in when it was taken out.

Then, when I inject it and try to get the result I want, I sometimes overcorrect it by about 5 or 10 percent. In other words, I build it up, knowing that some of the injected fat will not take and the area will go down.

Q: Do many Botox patients also have fat injections?
A: Yes. Many patients who have had Botox on their forehead find that they now look younger and feel better. The upper part of their faces now pleases them. But when they look at the lower part of their faces, they are troubled by

the area around the mouth, which may be sunken in and look old and lower. So that's where fat injections can help to revitalize the entire face.

Q: What is the difference in cost between fat injections and collagen?
A: If we were to do a procedure to fill out the smile folds with collagen, some patients would need between three and four syringes and each syringe would cost about $400. If we use fat for a similar procedure, the cost of six or eight syringes would be approximately the same price as three syringes of collagen, so using fat is very cost-effective for deep folds.

Q: Are there other advantages to using fat instead of collagen?
A: No skin test is required because you are getting your own fat. And fat, unlike implants (see below) or collagen, is very natural feeling. You don't really feel the substance in there, you just feel a fullness.

Q: How long do fat injections take to achieve their effect?
A: There is some swelling and it's better to plan to have them at least two full days before any big event—preferably four days, to be safe. The same is true for implants. Unlike implants, fat injections may be long-lasting, but cannot be considered permanent.

Q: What about the implants that you've mentioned? Are they like silicone?

A: Some newer products are being used for implants. Like silicone, they are fillers that are designed to plump up the wrinkles and lines, creating a smooth surface. For example, there is a permanent implant called UltraSoft, formerly called Softform, which is made of Gore-Tex. This synthetic material has been used not only in jackets to keep us warm and dry in the winter, but also, for over twenty-five years, by vascular surgeons for vein grafts.

Gore-Tex, consisting of solid threads or mesh, is a permanent implant and is used instead of fat or collagen, which are largely temporary. When Gore-Tex is implanted, the cosmetic effect usually looks very good.

Q: Are there any negative aspects to using Gore-Tex?

A: There is a downside: you can feel it. If you push your tongue against your cheek and touch your cheek on the outside with your fingers, you can feel the implanted tube, and you can even see it at times. But when you're at rest or even smiling, it is usually not apparent to others.

We can put this material into the lips as well. It does not resorb because it's a permanent item. If the patient isn't happy, it has to be surgically removed. Most surgeons won't charge for this removal, but if you are going to have another implant inserted, you will have to pay for that.

There is also a risk of infection, and once this occurs, the implant has to be removed. It will also have to be removed if it slides out of position or if the end becomes extruded from the skin.

Q: How much does this type of treatment cost?
A: These grafts are typically expensive. They could cost around $2,500 for two, one on each side. But if you have big smile folds, the price could be a lot more. However, these implants do work nicely for people who have big folds because if they take well and the people are happy with them, they don't have to keep coming back for more treatments, as they do with fat or collagen.

Q: Are companies working on any new fillers that might be better than the ones we have now?
A: There's a collagen product that is mixed with a glue. The glue remains as permanent particles and the collagen is used to deliver it wherever we want it to go. So as the collagen resorbs in the body, the glue material remains.

The concern with this product is that if someone has an allergic reaction, they could be troubled by long-term reactions, since the glue is not temporary, like ordinary collagen, and will not go away in six to nine months. So more investigation is needed on the development of this product.

Another exciting product in development is Isolagen, which is collagen made by fibroblasts. Fibroblasts are cells. The body makes collagen constantly, and if the skin is injured, it's healed from the bottom up, and then new skin comes in from the edges toward the middle. The collagen contributes to this healing process. Or when people have acne, the inflammation damages the undersurface and they get thinned-out areas with depressions or craters on the surface.

Collagen and silicone have been used in the past to fill up those craters. But now, by taking a small skin sample from behind your ear (to keep the scar hidden), and sending it to a laboratory, laboratories can grow fibroblasts for implantation. In other words, the lab is producing the cells that make your own collagen. These cells are then injected and planted in your skin.

Q: Then what happens?
A: You come back for several treatments, and over time there will be a buildup of new collagen that your body is producing. The acne scars will improve and fill out, which is actually quite amazing.

Q: When will this product be available?
A: The company is in their third phase of FDA studies, and it is also being investigated in Europe, so it might be a couple of years at most, if all goes well.

Q: What about surgical procedures to fill in areas?
A: There are surgical options, such as dermal grafts, in which doctors cut out some skin from behind the ear. They remove the epidermis then use the dermis, inserting it under the skin in an area where there's a depression, to help fill it up. But this is a more invasive procedure and is not in a class with the other fillers.

Q: Tell us about resurfacing procedures. What are they and what can they accomplish on the face?
A: Resurfacing can be used to improve lines that don't need to be filled out. The theory behind it is that if we

remove the topmost dead layer of the skin and go into the living layer below, the body will heal with new collagen and new skin that will grow out smoother. As a result, there will be fewer lines.

Q: How is the resurfacing done?
A: One way is to do it ablatively. That means we actually destroy the part we don't want, using lasers. Two other resurfacing methods are deep chemical peels and dermabrasion. The chemical peels cause blistering in order to make the skin shed its upper layer, while dermabrasion works by sanding away the outer layer of the skin.

Q: Can you give us more details about how the deep chemical peels work?
A: With deep chemical peels, we put a chemical on the skin that creates blistering. The blistering is equivalent to a second-degree burn. As the patient's skin heals over about a week and a half, newer skin grows and the collagen improves.

Q: What kinds of problems are helped by chemical peels?
A: These procedures can be used to treat dark spots, irregular skin tone, and moderate lines.

Q: What about the lighter peels, like the ones you can get in a doctor's office or beauty parlor?
A: They are not the same at all. Some of the lighter peels

done in a doctor's office are superficial, and are used for very mild lines. They may cause your skin to flake, much like it does after a sunburn, or in some cases, the skin may not flake at all, but it does not blister. The healing time for these lighter peels is sometimes only one day.

There is an even lighter type of peel done by a cosmetologist, aesthetician, or sometimes by nurses and physicians. I call it a "superficial superficial peel." It is very mild and only creates a little flaking, sometimes none at all. These are the true lunchtime peels.

Q: What are the ingredients in these "superficial superficial" peels?
A: They use mild alpha hydroxy acids, the fruit acids found in so many cosmetic products. Depending on their strength, these acids can improve the sheen and texture of the skin, and sometimes its coloration, and they also help other creams to penetrate better. But they will not erase moderate lines and probably will not affect the mild lines, either.

Q: What do alpha hydroxy acids actually do for the skin?
A: In the cosmetic products you buy over-the-counter, they are very mild exfoliants and can remove some of the dead skin on the uppermost layer. But the alpha hydroxy acids used by physicians and in deeper chemical peels are more concentrated. They will reach deeper into the skin and encourage the production of new cells and new col-

lagen, helping to smooth mild lines and some skin discoloration.

Most of these products say they contain "natural fruit acids," but in reality, the ingredients are synthesized in a laboratory. Even in low concentrations, these acids will feel tingly and can cause the skin to become red, a side effect that usually goes away after a few hours.

Q: So there are different depths of peels and you need to know which is appropriate for you?
A: That's right. The depth is directly proportional to the amount of improvement you want. And it's also directly proportional to the amount of risk you feel comfortable taking.

Q: What are the risks of the medium peels?
A: There are risks of scarring, developing wounds that don't heal, or having long-term redness or permanent lightness on the face. We don't tend to have problems with whiteness unless a deep peel is used, but there can be discoloration with blotches of darkened skin.

Q: What other options exist for resurfacing and improving the look of the facial skin?
A: Another useful process is dermabrasion. It is performed with a mechanical, rotary device that uses a diamond wheel or a wire brush to thoroughly strip away the epidermis and get down to deeper layers. However, you are left with a bloody surface that has to heal. That can take about ten or more days of downtime.

Q: What about lasers? Have they been used for re-surfacing for a long time?

A: Lasers have been used for surgery for many years. There have been many different types of lasers over the years. One of the first lasers used for resurfacing the face was the carbon dioxide, or CO_2 laser. At first, it seemed very effective and we were pleased with the results.

Q: How does the CO_2 laser work?

A: A carbon-dioxide laser vaporizes off the top layer of skin by using heat, and in so doing it also creates heat damage, like a mild burn. The idea is that this mild burn helps to initiate some tightening of the skin and will produce more collagen when the skin grows back and heals.

Q: Are there problems with lasers?

A: As with almost anything, there are some unwanted side effects. With the CO_2 laser, we discovered that about a year after treatment, some patients developed a delayed hypopigmentation, or lightening of the skin, that is permanent. With lasers, as with all types of resurfacing procedures, there is also a risk of scarring. This can also happen with dermabrasion, chemical peels, and laser resurfacing. Redness is also a common side effect with lasers. We found that some people have redness around the eyes for many months after laser surgery and they have to camouflage it with makeup.

So a new type of laser has been developed. It's called the Erbium Yag and is much gentler and less destructive per pass (a single use) than the CO_2 laser.

Q: So is the Erbium Yag now the laser of the first choice?
A: It isn't perfect. The Erbium Yag does not remove as much skin, so you need to make more passes to get the same effect as the CO_2 laser. But you don't have the thermal, or heat, side effect that you get with the CO_2. Because of this, the Erbium Yag can remove just the surface. Your skin heals a little faster than with the CO_2, but the Erbium Yag doesn't seem to create the same tightening effect. But it does create less intense redness, and that redness goes away much faster than it does with the CO_2.

Q: Are there any other types of lasers being used for resurfacing?
A: There is a newer generation, developed within about the past five or six years. One of them incorporates features of both the CO_2 and the Erbium Yag, and another one uses an Erbium Yag with a longer pulse duration, meaning that the fraction of a second that the laser strikes the skin is longer. Both allow quicker healing than the CO_2 and still allow for some tightening effect.

Q: Do many people have laser resurfacing?
A: Because of the possibility of so many unwanted side effects, including persistent redness, the risk of scarring, and the downtime, many people have decided not to have laser resurfacing in the past few years.

But the interesting thing is that we now have a modified version of an old workhorse, the Pulsed Dye laser, which has been used since the early 1980s for infants and chil-

dren with congenital red birthmarks, the port wine stains.
This new laser is called the "V" Beam. It can be used for
noninvasive, nonablative photo-rejuvenation. Other nonablative lasers include the Cool-Touch, Smooth Beam,
and N-Lite.

Q: How do nonablative lasers work?
A: These lasers do not open the skin, so there is no bleeding. They may cause slight redness and swelling, but not
a wound. The laser beams are going through the skin and
being absorbed by our tiny capillaries or blood vessels.
These beams also produce a heat effect, but it's produced
deep down below, where it stimulates the production of
collagen.

Using this type of laser, we can treat mild lines around
the eyes, and even some lines around the lips, and it only
creates a little redness that goes away within a few hours.
Then, over successive treatments, usually one to two
months apart, the lines are improved by the newer collagen building up underneath the skin.

Q: What about the results?
A: They are not as great as laser resurfacing, deep chemical peels, or dermabrasion, but if patients can't afford the
downtime, the nonablative lasers may be their best choice.

Q: Are there any other alternatives for improving fa-
cial skin?
A: Yes. Another treatment is cryotherapy. It involves

freezing the skin, using liquid nitrogen that is a few hundred degrees below zero, to create blistering. Cryotherapy is usually used to peel off precancers on the face. But it has also been used by physicians on the entire face to shed layers of skin, so it is comparable to laser resurfacing and dermabrasion.

Dermasanding is another treatment that is similar to dermabrasion, but instead of a rotary device, it involves the use of a block of sterilized sandpaper. This sandpaper rubs the wrinkles raw and is sometimes used in conjunction with other treatments.

Coblation is yet another newer treatment. It uses an electrical current and a conductive liquid medium, such as saline solution. The electrode is passed very close to the skin and the current goes through the saline (or other) liquid and into the skin. This procedure stimulates the skin to make new collagen. But coblation also lifts off the skin surface and causes wounds, so it is similar to the CO_2 laser, requiring several days to heal.

Q: Is there a way to improve the surface of the skin without all the potential unwanted side effects, such as bruising, redness, wounding, and even scarring?
A: There certainly are far less irritating methods available, but in most cases, they do not achieve results that are as good. But you can combine some of the topical products, such as alpha hydroxy acids, Retin-A, Kinerase (which is a plant derivative), vitamin E, vitamin C, and other antioxidants with, perhaps, a nonablative laser and maybe a few microdermabrasion treatments—the gentle form—and get pretty good results.

Q: We've heard so much about Retin-A. Can you tell us a little about it?
A: The active ingredient in Retin-A is tretinoin, an extract of vitamin A. Retin-A has been used for many years to treat acne. It also helps reverse photo-damage from the sun, making the skin smoother, causing fine lines to fade or disappear, and giving you a more youthful appearance. Retin-A also appears to increase collagen production in the skin and minimize the formation of new precancers on the face.

You have to be extremely careful about sun exposure when using Retin-A because the ingredients make you more sun-sensitive. So you must use sunscreen faithfully. Retin-A does not work for everyone and can also cause irritation of the skin surface. Many people's facial skin can become accustomed to this, but a few cannot.

Q: It seems that combining products and treatments can often be helpful for various types of skin problems. Do many people have combinations of treatments?
A: Combination treatment has become much more the norm today. That's why it is so important to have a complete evaluation by a qualified physician. In that way, an individualized program can be formulated to deal with your unique face and skin, and what you want to achieve.

Q: What about sagging jowls or cheeks? What can be done for them?
A: Sagging jowls don't always mean you have to have a face-lift, but it is often the best way to solve the problem.

Unlike smile folds, which frequently do not respond to face-lifts, jowls are liftable.

But there are different degrees of sagging jowls, and if they are not severe, we can smooth down the area with neck liposuction. So instead of an expensive and invasive face-lift, patients only have small nicks in their skin underneath the chin, visible only to their shoe salesperson or podiatrist.

Q: What do you look for when you evaluate patients?
A: I look at their faces, find out which areas concern them, and try to determine whether they have superficial, medium, or deep skin problems. If patients ask me to treat just one spot, I don't tell them, "By the way, you're also damaged here and there and you need these other treatments."

But if they ask me, "What can you recommend to make my face look younger overall?" then I will review the whole list. I start from the top and go to the bottom, from the forehead to the chin and neck. Then I go from superficial to deep, asking myself, "Is it coloration? Is it splotchy brown? Is it splotchy white? Is it a chronic sundamage sallowness?"

Then I evaluate the lines on the face. Are they very fine, moderate, or deep? Next I look at the cosmetic units between the lines, not just the smile folds and crow's-feet, but between the two, the midcheek area. Is there any cross-hatching? Is there cobblestoning? Lines can become very deep, and instead of just lines, the grooves form almost squares or diamonds and the skin between them outpockets and protrudes, and has a sallow color. So there can be yellow diagonal bumps on the cheek.

Q: What about youthfulness or lack of it in the skin?
A: I look at the elasticity of the skin, and how much of it has been lost. I also examine the blood vessels on the face. Many patients say, "I want to look better and I want fewer wrinkles, but I also want you to treat those blood vessels in my face so it won't be so red."

Normally, I tell these people, "When we treat your lines and your skin texture, there is a very good chance that while you're healing, you are going to be redder. So let's not waste your money and treat your redness twice. Let's start by doing the resurfacing technique, and once you've healed, if there is still any redness left over, we can treat it then." And we treat it with the same laser we use for noninvasive facial rejuvenation without any bruising.

So you see, there are many different types of treatments and many different combinations that can be tailored to each individual for maximum improvement of whatever skin problems are bothering them. Today, Botox is the number one choice for most people who want more youthful-looking skin, but Botox cannot do everything, and it is often one part of a group of treatments that together can yield wonderful results.

To Summarize:

- There are other products similar to Botox, but so far, Botox appears the best choice for the problems and the areas it treats.

- Collagen, derived from cows, has been used for some time as an injected filler for facial lines and creases. Treatments must be repeated every four to six months, and it can be used in combination with Botox or in areas where Botox can't be used.

- Other fillers include silicone (rarely used today), which is a permanent implant; Hylaform, Restylane, and Perlane, which may soon be approved by the FDA.

- Smile folds can be treated with collagen or with fat injections, derived from the patient's own fat.

- After using Botox on the upper part of the face, many people have fat injections on the lower half of the face in order to revitalize the entire face.

- Newer implant products can be cost-effective over time and can plump up facial wrinkles and lines, creating a smooth surface.

- Pharmaceutical companies are working on developing more effective treatments, some using recombinant DNA.

- For some people, plastic surgery can provide the best results.

- The appearance of the skin can be improved by resurfacing techniques, including deep chemical peels, dermabrasion, and laser treatments.

- All these treatments have some risk of unwanted side effects, including redness, lightening, irregular darkening of the skin, and scarring.

- Topical products applied directly to the skin include alpha hydroxy acids, Retin-A, Kinerase, and vitamins C and E in creams and lotions. All can obtain good results and make the skin smoother and more youthful looking with long-term use.

- Most patients have combination treatments, which include Botox and one or more of the other approaches.

Chapter 9

Dr. Shelton's Lifelong Program for Healthy,
Youthful Skin

We have seen how many different treatments and products can help you rejuvenate your skin and make you look much younger and more attractive. Although Botox is one of the most effective, there are others that can be used in combination with Botox or for areas and problems that Botox cannot treat.

But when it comes to having and maintaining young, healthy skin, the most important factor of all is prevention. From the time we are born, our skin can be damaged in many different ways. If we begin a prevention program early and do all the right things, our chances of keeping supple and young-looking skin will be greatly enhanced.

To begin, let's look at Dr. Shelton's acronym for better skin:

N — No smoking

I — Injections: Botox, collagen, fat

C — Cleansers

E — Exfoliation: microdermabrasion and chemical
      peels

F — Facial laser noninvasive rejuvenation and flu-
      ids (hydration)

A — Alpha hydroxy acids and vitamin A

C — Vitamin C creams and lotions

E — Emollients: Kinerase

S — Sunscreen, sleep

This acronym, NICE FACES, will help you to remember
some of the most critical factors for achieving and maintaining youthful, healthy skin. Let's look at them in more
detail.

PART ONE:
YOUR SELF-HELP PROGRAM

**Q: What are the three most important things women
and men can do to take care of their skin and prevent
the signs of aging?**
A: They are, literally, in this order: (1) sunscreen; (2)
sunscreen; and (3) sunscreen. And I'm being serious.

Q: And after sunscreen?
A: (4) no smoking; (5) Retin-A; (6) a healthy diet; (7)
good hydration with water; (8) no hot water on the skin,

just lukewarm; (9) moisturizers; (10) alpha hydroxy or fruit acids; (11) vitamin C creams and lotions; (12) low to moderate alcohol consumption; (13) sufficient rest and sleep. That would be it for about 90 percent of people.

Q: Let's talk first about the things people can do on their own, without a doctor. You mention sunscreen as being, by far, the single most important factor in skin protection. Does that also include avoiding sun-tanning parlors, which are so popular today, especially with young people?

A: The major cause of an aging face is, without a doubt, sun damage. Remember that a person with a lot of facial wrinkles has only to look at the underside of the upper arm to see how the skin there, which has not been exposed to the sun, has retained its normal color and smoothness. It may have very fine lines and some loss of elasticity, but it doesn't have the deep grooves we find on the face.

So sunscreen is critically important, and by sunscreen, we also include other sun protection techniques, such as wearing sunglasses and a wide-brimmed hat, staying out of the midday sun when the rays are strongest, and avoiding intentionally getting a suntan.

Staying away from suntan parlors is certainly included here, because when the skin turns brown from ultraviolet rays, it's a sign of radiation damage, and those signs are going to come back to haunt you later in the form of wrinkles, lines, and other damage to your skin.

If people are really intent on getting a bronzed look, they should stay away from suntan parlors and instead do it artificially with tanning lotions and salon-spraying treatments, which tend to give a more uniform, less streaky appearance, all without the dangers of ultraviolet-ray exposure.

Q: Are these artificial tanning methods harmful to the skin in any way?
A: No, because they are based on an inert pigment that is only deposited in the outer dead layer of skin. So as we naturally exfoliate day by day, the treatments lose their intensity. And, of course, there can be no DNA damage if the product only reaches the dead layer of the epidermis.

Am I promoting these artificial tans? No, I'm not. But I am realistic enough to know that if people really want a darker skin color, especially if they have had skin cancer, it would be far better for them to apply a spray than to go to the beach or suntan parlor.

Q: What about protecting the skin on your arms, legs, and other parts of your body that may be exposed in warm weather?
A: Interestingly enough, if you are outside in warm weather, long-sleeved shirts will not only protect your skin, they will also keep you cooler than short-sleeved shirts, especially when the sun is beating down on you.

If you have concerns about sun damage on your hands, put sunscreen on them. Some people even wear white cotton gloves when they drive just to provide further protection to their skin.

The sunscreen you use should have a minimum SPF (sun protection factor) of 15 and should also be waterproof, if you are going to perspire or go swimming. If you plan to be in direct sunlight, increase the SPF and reapply the sunscreen every hour. It's also a good idea to apply your sunscreen about thirty minutes before you go outside so it can bind better to the skin.

Q: What about the influence of the food we eat on our skin? What are some preventive steps we can take with diet before the skin is damaged?

A: Diet is another important consideration, something that we need to maintain throughout our lives. If we eat a balanced diet that contains enough protein, the skin will certainly benefit.

Protein is also important for healthy collagen, and a protein deficiency will definitely slow down normal collagen production in the skin.

It's also important to warn people not to go on a no-fat diet. So many foods today have labels reading "no fat" or "low fat," and some treats even have a synthetic chemical that tastes like fat. If people consume only these products and avoid all other fats, they could end up being deficient in essential fatty acids, which are actually very important for healthy skin and other organs in the body. People who are deficient in fatty acids can develop a dermatitis or an inflammatory skin condition that creates redness, peeling, and oozing.

Q: How much fat do we need each day?

A: Approximately one-third of your calories during the day should come from fat, but it should be polyunsaturated fat. Some experts suggest a lower percentage, about

20 percent of daily calories. We should especially try to consume the alpha omega fatty acids that are found in many fish such as salmon, and some people should add vitamin supplements to get the amounts they need. Fat should not be avoided altogether, but the fat we consume must be the healthier type, not the saturated type.

You have to watch what you eat and see how much of your intake is coming from fat, how much from carbohydrates, and how much from protein—you need all three. You can't be healthy by eating only carbohydrates or only protein.

Q: How can you know exactly what diet is right for you?
A: It's a good idea to consult your physician or nutritionist rather than just believe what you hear or read in the latest bestseller.

Q: What about drinking water and other fluids?
A: Hydration is extremely important for healthy skin. If people are not drinking enough during the day, their kidneys are still excreting what they need to excrete, but in a more concentrated form. If they continue like this for a while, they can run the risk of eventually having their kidneys begin to fail. And if the by-products of protein increase in the blood because the kidneys are not working well, the skin will be affected.

You have to remember that skin is composed significantly of water, in the ground substance that we mentioned earlier. And if people become dehydrated, the elasticity of the skin is affected—it just doesn't bounce back the way it should.

Q: What else happens to the skin as a result of de-hydration?
A: Your skin gets thinner, you develop more wrinkles, and you have a loss of moisture and elasticity. Remember that we talked about the skin's turgor, its fullness and firmness. Dehydration causes the skin to sag all over, and that will give you a very haggard and aged appearance.

Q: How much water do people need every day?
A: We have all heard that people should drink eight eight-ounce glasses of water a day, but it's really an individual thing. It could be a quart of water a day when you add up all the other beverages we tend to drink. With a quart of water, most healthy people will do well, provided they are drinking other beneficial fluids. But you can't really hurt yourself by drinking more. Your kidneys will process it.

However, if you have certain diseases, like congestive heart failure, that's a different story. So it's always best to check with your doctor about proper fluid consumption for your individual body.

Q: What about people who don't like to drink plain water?
A: You have to realize that if you don't like to drink water, you can't simply make up for it by drinking soda or coffee. If the beverage has caffeine, which is a diuretic,

it will make you excrete more water in your urine than you normally would, so the liquid is not hydrating your body as well as noncaffeinated beverages. In other words, if you drink only caffeinated liquids, you can actually go into a negative balance and do yourself harm.

Q: So would you say that caffeine is bad for your skin?
A: It should be used in moderation. If someone is drinking caffeinated beverages all day long, they won't be hydrating their skin as effectively as if they are drinking water.

Q: What about smoking? That was pretty high up on your list.
A: Smoke is composed of chemicals that are known to be toxic. So when people smoke, there is a systemic toxicity throughout the bloodstream. The same thing happens with the secondhand smoke you inhale either from other people smoking or from your own smoking.

People talk about secondhand smoke and always think about the smoker next to them. But smokers themselves are inhaling smoke through their lungs from the cigarette and then they are also inhaling the smoke they blow out, through their noses. So they're actually breathing the smoke twice, one time intentionally and the other time not.

Q: What does that double intake of smoke do?
A: It depletes the skin and the whole body of oxygen.

That means that the oxygen, which should be going through your bloodstream, is interrupted and lessened. If your body is not saturated with oxygen, then your turnover of new skin cells won't work as well, they won't be as efficient.

So the toxic chemicals in the smoke, plus the lack of proper oxygen, will combine to damage the skin and create the prematurely aged appearance that we see in so many heavy smokers.

Q: What about the effects of alcohol on the skin?
A: Significant alcohol consumption dehydrates the skin and diminishes the amount of important vitamins that the skin can acquire. Some people develop vitamin B_{12} deficiencies, and they can even lead to the deficiency disease pellagra, in which the skin can look very aged.

But we are not talking about an occasional glass of wine or a few beers or a hard drink from time to time. We are talking about significant drinking over a long period of time.

Q: Why are rest and relaxation beneficial for our skin?
A: Because they counteract stress. Stress adds lines to the face because of tension and the facial grimacing that results from tension. Very often, you don't even realize you are grimacing and stressing your skin.

When most people come back from a vacation, they usually hear people say, "You look so good!" It doesn't necessarily mean that they have a tan (we hope they don't), but that they don't have that stern face with the muscles clenched in a constant position of anger or tension—the clenched expression that creates more and deeper lines on your face.

Stress can also be a result of your emotional state. If you are angry, depressed, or worried about something, your facial expressions can contribute to skin damage.

Q: How much sleep do we need?
A: Enough so that you feel alert and well rested. For some people, that means eight hours a night, while for others it can be seven hours or less.

Sleep is needed to lower the basal metabolic rate. If you are metabolizing things rapidly and you're constantly metabolizing, you become very hyper. Every minute of the day and night you are doing five things at the same time, and by doing that, you are also creating harmful by-products of metabolism.

Every cell that's living in your body needs nutrients, oxygen, and water, and then it has by-products. When you're sleeping at night and your basal metabolic rate goes down, you produce fewer of these by-products.

The body is designed to get rid of certain by-products at a specific rate, and there's a potential that too much activity on a long-term basis will create an excess of these by-products, including the free radicals that we've discussed, which will increase and do more damage.

So a good night's sleep and rest are as important to healthy skin as sunscreen protection, not smoking, and the other components we've discussed.

Q: What is your opinion about vitamin supplements? Can they help to keep our skin younger?

A: There is still a great deal we need to learn about nutritional supplements. Many people will do fine with a well-balanced diet. Taking supplements and having more of a vitamin or mineral does not necessarily mean that it's going to improve your health or appearance.

If you are deficient in vitamin C and you take a vitamin C supplement, you will get improvement in the problems that are caused by a deficiency, but if you are not deficient and you take a lot of vitamin C, it doesn't mean that you will become younger looking.

Scientists are still studying the effects of supplementation, trying to design controlled studies that will eliminate all the variables and test for one thing at a time. So we will have to wait for better scientific evidence.

Q: Vitamin C was on your list of items that benefit the skin. What form of vitamin C are you recommending?
A: I am recommending the topical form of vitamin C that is available in some skin products. Vitamin C is an antioxidant, and when it is used in specially made creams and lotions, it goes directly into the skin and appears to have some sun protection properties.

Q: Where can you buy these products?
A: There are many over-the-counter products that contain vitamin C, but only a very few companies know how to make their vitamin C stable. That's why it is best to get a vitamin C product that is recommended and usually dispensed by a dermatologist or plastic surgeon.

Q: What about using only lukewarm water and not hot water on your skin? Why is that important?
A: Hot water is going to take the oils right out of your skin much more than lukewarm water would. Hot water will start to dry you out. So lukewarm water is all you really need, and then, if you tend to have slightly dry skin, you should put on a moisturizer very soon after washing your face. That will lock in the moisture and also avoid other problems.

Q: What kinds of problems?
A: Some people get eczema, an inflammatory condition related to dryness, which could be avoided by using moisturizers on damp skin to trap the water in the skin and not let it evaporate.

Q: If hot water isn't good for your skin, then what about steam? Are saunas or steam baths or even those hot steamy towels you get in Japanese restaurants bad for your skin?
A: Steam is a fine moisturizer for the skin, as long as you put on a moisturizing cream or lotion immediately afterward. Otherwise, the hot water in the steam will draw the moisture out of your skin and end up evaporating and drying it out, defeating your purpose.

Q: What about cleansers? Should people ever use soap on their faces?
A: Dove soap, which is about one-quarter moisturizing lotion, is a nonirritating soap that can be safely used by

most people. People should be very careful to use only nonirritating cleansers. Some people have used only one product for many years and are doing well with it, so I would usually not recommend any changes for them.

But if someone complains of dry skin or combination skin or irritated skin, they should use a nonirritating cleanser like Cetaphil, which is an over-the-counter product. There is a type of Cetaphil for oily skin as well. Neutrogena also has a cleanser for dry skin, as do other companies.

Q: What moisturizers can you recommend?
A: When it comes to moisturizers, many work well. Good old Vaseline around the eyelids can do wonders. But some people react to the greasier component and prefer a finer cream, especially during the daytime.

Cetaphil, which is a cleanser, can also serve as a moisturizer. Eucerin is another good facial moisturizer, as is Moisturel. There are also special nonprescription products that you can find in a doctor's office, especially for people with very sensitive skin, such as Tolerin, the line made by LaRoche Posay.

Q: Are the commercial masques that so many cosmetic companies sell actually good for your skin? Do they deep-clean the pores and remove debris or can they have negative effects?
A: Each of these masques is made differently and has different ingredients, so we can't generalize about them. Some can be too drying by drawing out a lot of moisture

in the skin, so you have to put on your moisturizer right afterward.

Q: We are exposed to so much pollution and dirt. How do you know when your face is really clean?
A: Some people are rightly concerned about the effects of environmental pollution on the skin. Especially in large cities and industrial areas, the skin can really take a beating from all the irritants to which we are constantly exposed. So you do want to clean your face sufficiently to remove these pollutants.

Even so, you don't want to overclean, because as we said earlier, if you scrub your face more than three times a day, you can stimulate more oil production and get into a catch-22 situation. You can also cause a problem with overexfoliation, where too much of the surface of your skin is being stripped away.

If you keep scrubbing your face and then add alpha hydroxy acid products or Retin-A or have microdermabrasion treatments or use cleansers with granules constantly, you will take away the protective barrier so much that you can develop chronic sensitivity syndrome, in which almost anything you put on your face burns and irritates your skin.

So moderation is the key. Wash your face with lukewarm water and a nonirritating cleanser no more than two or three times a day.

Q: Do you have to use soap or a cleanser to clean your face?
A: There are many women who wash their faces with

water only, and for them, it works. I don't tell them to change, because I can see that their results are good and their skin is clean and healthy.

But the average person needs something more to clean away the surface oils and keep the pores clear of debris. As you recall, we shed dead skin all the time and the skin cells near the pores can accumulate, creating a fertile ground for the growth of bacteria.

When this happens, you start to have a lot of bacteria growing in the pores and combining with the oils. The bacteria break down the oils into inflammation-provoking fatty acids, which can end up as acne.

But if you use a gentle cleanser that does not harm the skin, it will also help decrease problems with skin break-outs. Of course, if acne or other serious problems do develop, medical treatment may be necessary.

Q: Are toners useful?
A: Not really. You have to realize that even if a toner feels good on your skin, its effects last for about fifteen seconds. Toners do shrink the pores temporarily, and if people like them, they can continue using them, but they are really not that effective.

Most toners are made from alcohol or propylene glycol (an alcohol derivative), and these substances are rather caustic to the skin. They strip the oils from our layers. So a toner might give you a nice, astringent feeling, but most people should not use it more than once a day.

There are some people with very oily skin who can tolerate greater use, and again, if it works for them, fine. But if they start to develop eczema or inflammation, they may have to stop using toners.

It's simply not a good idea to buy any astringent you like and use it to clean your face five times a day. That will not be good for your skin.

Q: What other things that we do can damage the skin?
A: Scrubbing hard with a washcloth, picking at the pores or picking at acne can all be very harmful. These things put the skin at risk. Bursting the sac of debris and the sac of skin cells that are growing below the skin surface can create significant inflammation that can even result in facial scarring.

Q: What about physical exercise? Is it good for the skin?
A: While the exercise itself may be beneficial, outdoor exercise does present a risk of sun exposure. People who are devoted athletes and spend a lot of time exercising outdoors will often get very leathery skin, even if they use lots of sunscreen.

You have to remember that when you are exercising outside, you are also perspiring and that can quickly dilute the sunscreen. So even if you take precautions, your skin will receive damaging sun exposure. Reapply the sunscreen often in this case in order to avoid a sunburn.

Of course, there are people who are so devoted to their sports that they are willing to put up with the skin problems. They know it's a risky situation and they take all the precautions they can, but they are not going to give up their tennis or golf or swimming, even after they develop skin cancers.

Q: Aside from possible sun damage, are all types of exercise good for the skin?
A: Not necessarily. Many forms of exercise can dry out the skin, including running, jogging in the winter, snowboarding, ice skating, and skiing. You can put on moisturizer and a mask for these sports and this will give your skin some protection.

Many people who engage in these sports notice that they have flakes of skin on their faces and chapping on their lips during the drier seasons when there is less moisture in the air. So it's important to use a sunscreen that also serves as a moisturizer, especially waterproof sunscreens, because they trap in the water.

Q: So you can have two products in one, a sunscreen and a moisturizer?
A: Yes. Sunscreens can act as moisturizers. But it's important to know that the reverse is not true. Moisturizers with a sunscreen ingredient do not act well as sunscreens themselves. They just aren't as effective as the sunscreens because of the much lower concentration of the sunscreening ingredients.

You also have to experiment to find the sunscreen that works best for you. It's really trial and error. Some of them are too greasy and some migrate and sting the eyes. Coppertone Sport is one product that does not tend to burn the eyes; products that have been micronized, and contain small bits of titanium dioxide or zinc oxide, are also good. It's a good idea to try any new sunscreen product on a little patch of skin first to be certain that you don't have a reaction to it.

Q: What about our facial expressions? We know that lines and wrinkles come from using our muscles over the years to make certain expressions. Can we minimize wrinkling by changing these expressions?
A: If you are very concerned about having creases, then you might think about doing this. If you're worried about having forehead creases, you might not want to look overly surprised or exaggerate your expressions. In addition, you should use sunglasses to avoid squinting. If you're worried about creases between your brows, you should develop an awareness of whether you are frowning without realizing it, as many people do throughout the day, especially at work when they are concentrating.

Some people have a habit of sneering a bit when they talk, again without realizing it. One side of the mouth comes out more than the other side, and eventually they develop more of a smile groove on that side of the face.

Q: How can you become more aware of these damaging facial expressions?
A: In most cases, someone needs to point them out. This typically happens during a consultation in the doctor's office. The doctor may give these patients a mirror and ask them to talk or respond and then observe what they are doing with their faces. This can make them more conscious of what they are doing.

Then, when they are talking to someone, they may begin to realize, "Gosh, my eyebrow just went up. When I'm a little tense or stern and I'm questioning someone, my left eyebrow comes way up high, and now I feel it." They may then go to a mirror and look to see what is going on. Then the next time it happens, they will start to feel the muscle move and they will control it.

Of course, you can go to a mirror and try to see these things for yourself, but it often takes an outside observer to point them out to you.

Q: What other things that we do without realizing it can cause facial lines?
A: If you are really interested in preserving a youthful appearance, you should try to sleep on your back if possible. When you sleep on your side, there is a chance that you will develop what we call a "sleep crease," which is a groove, usually vertical to somewhat diagonal along the temple. Since these creases are not muscle-related, Botox can't help them. You can put collagen in them, but it's much cheaper and easier to try to sleep on your back and avoid creating them in the first place.

Q: But people don't sleep in one position all night, do they?
A: Yes, that's correct. You do tend to roll over in your sleep and many people say they are not comfortable sleeping on their backs. Or perhaps their mattresses are sagging and need to be replaced.

If you remind yourself when you first go to sleep that you want to lie on your back and keep your skin smooth, it might influence your sleep patterns and you might begin to find the position more comfortable.

Q: What about facial exercises? Are they good for your skin?

A: The jury is still out on this. Many years ago, some doctors advocated such exercises, thinking they would help tone or strengthen facial muscles. But there is still no definitive proof that they are beneficial.

Of course, it depends on exactly what kind of facial exercises you are doing. If the exercises pull the cheek inward, you may see your smile folds deepen. Anything that repetitively puts the skin in a crease is eventually going to make that crease permanent. So there is a possibility that, like certain facial expressions, these exercises may help to create lines rather than avoid them.

There are also electric stimulators that are thought to help smooth out lines and we don't think they are harmful. We don't know if it's actually the electric stimulation that makes the lines look better. It's possible that the electric stimulation could be creating new collagen underneath the skin, similar to noninvasive laser rejuvenation. This technique has not been studied enough to know if it's truly clinically effective.

Q: Can yo-yo dieting, where you lose and gain and lose and gain weight repeatedly, damage your skin?
A: Dieting of this kind can definitely stress the body. When people are dieting, their bodies contain more by-products, more free radicals, to damage the skin.

It also depends on what diet you are following. If you are on a low-carbohydrate diet, your body gets energy by converting proteins. The carbohydrates that we consume get stored as both fat and glycogen in the liver. When carbohydrates are diminished, we start to convert the glycogen, but we soon run out of it and then it takes a longer time to burn fat. The body needs energy, so it then starts to deplete stores of protein and decrease muscle mass.

The infrastructure of the skin is made of protein and the blood vessel wall is made of protein. As you become deficient, you begin to lose the strength of the skin. You will start to bruise more easily and the texture underneath will start to thin out. The skin begins to take on a more fragile appearance and it may tear more easily and not heal as well.

So yes, yo-yo dieting can add stress not only to the skin, but also to the internal organs. It is not healthy, and if done to extreme, over and over, it can create very serious problems, not only for the skin, but for the entire body.

To Summarize:

- Using sunscreen is the single most important way to prevent aging skin. Wearing sunglasses and a wide-brimmed hat and avoiding the midday sun are also important.

- Other preventive measures include no smoking, use of Retin-A, a good diet, good liquid intake, no hot water on the skin, use of moisturizers, alpha hydroxy acids and special vitamin C lotions and creams, low to moderate alcohol consumption, and sufficient rest and sleep.

- Avoid suntan parlors, which cause the skin to age and to produce wrinkles. Use tanning lotions instead, if you must.

- The skin needs fat to be healthy. In its polyunsaturated form, fat should be included in your everyday diet.

- Lack of proper hydration contributes to wrinkling and loss of skin elasticity. Consume at least a quart of water every day and more if possible, along with other fluids, unless your doctor tells you otherwise. Avoid too many beverages with caffeine.

- Avoid smoking and secondhand smoke, which depletes the body of oxygen, prematurely drying out and aging the skin.

- Heavy alcohol consumption dehydrates skin, contributing to wrinkles.

- Proper rest and sleep help avoid stress and tension and the accompanying facial expressions that age the skin.

- Bathing too often or using hot water and rough cleansers can deplete natural oils or cause their overproduction, damaging the skin.

- Some outdoor activities can damage skin.

- Some habitual facial expressions contribute to unwanted lines on the face.

PART TWO:
YOUR MEDICAL PROGRAM

We have covered many of the things you can do on your own to protect your skin and keep it supple and youthful—or at the very least, avoid any further damage. But there are additional options available to people who work with a physician, usually a dermatologist, to protect and improve their skin. Let's look at some of them.

Q: Should everyone go to a dermatologist? If so, when and how often?
A: Not everyone should go to a dermatologist. However, if you observe significant signs of aging, or if you have a suspicion that there's a spot on your skin that doesn't seem normal, or the color of your skin is changing and it concerns you, then you should definitely go.

In addition, products such as Retin-A require a doctor's prescription, and doctors can also make further recommendations for treatment, so seeing a dermatologist is important for some people.

I believe that a board-certified dermatologist is the best-trained doctor to determine what is and what is not malignant on the skin. But I certainly respect, and am grateful to, many of my nondermatologist colleagues, whether they are doctors in family practice, internal medicine, plastic surgery, or dentists and beauticians, who have referred patients appropriately.

Q: What are some of the reasons for consulting a dermatologist?
A: If you have a family member with a history of skin cancer, it is a very good idea to have yourself checked out. If you were born with a lot of moles on your skin— some people have fifty or even a hundred red-brown moles, sometimes as large as a quarter, all over their backs

and chests, for example—you should at least have a base-line examination.

If you are interested in treatment for acne, psoriasis, problems with your hair or nails, or general skin problems such as dermatitis, you should see a dermatologist.

Q: What about cosmetic concerns?
A: Yes, of course. Even if you don't have any medical concerns, but you are interested in improving the aged appearance of your skin, you should consult a dermatologist to find out what kind of treatments are available for you. You can also see an aesthetician or a cosmetologist, but seeing a dermatologist gives you many more options.

Q: What are some of the prescription medications that a dermatologist might recommend to treat specific problems or help people take good care of their skin?
A: One of the most commonly prescribed is vitamin A cream. There are several brands. As we have already mentioned, the chemical name is tretinoin and it is marketed under such brand names as Retin-A, Retin-A Micro, Renova, Differin, and Avita. These products come in cream, gel, and liquid forms. All are in the vitamin A family.

When Retin-A first came out, some people found it to be a little harsh on their skin. It wasn't a true drying effect, but it did produce some scaling and redness. In most cases, the skin gets used to it after a while, but the manufacturers have also created different formulas that are gentler and can be used by people with more sensitive skin.

Q: What does Retin-A do?
A: Retin-A is used to help reverse some kinds of damage from sun exposure. It can improve the unevenness of skin tone for people who have little bits of blotchy, brown coloring. It can also improve the luster or the blush of the skin by helping to regenerate some of the superficial capillaries or blood vessels in the skin that affect circulation.

Retin-A also improves the damaged collagen below the epidermis. Studies that examined skin under microscopes have proven that long-term use of Retin-A will actually minimize some of the damage from extended sun exposure. Retin-A makes the surface of the skin smoother, evens out the skin tone, and improves the skin's tensile strength. In fact, it improves the overall resiliency of the skin by improving the collagen underneath.

Q: Does Retin-A help with lines and wrinkles on the face?
A: It can minimize some fine lines, but it does not make moderate or deep lines go away. Nor does it remove the cobblestoning or crosshatch marks on the cheeks. But it definitely improves luster and some of the fine lines.

Q: How long do you have to use Retin-A to get these effects?
A: You really need to use it consistently for years, not for weeks or months.

Q: Since the active ingredient in Retin-A and similar products is a form of vitamin A, will taking vitamin A supplements have similar results?

A: Vitamin A, taken orally in high doses, can actually be quite dangerous. It is toxic to the pancreas, liver, and bones and can cause night-vision problems, excessively dry and peeling skin, and sometimes bleeding around the corners of the mouth, the lips, and the fingers. So like vitamin C, vitamin A is most effective on the skin in topical preparations like Retin-A, not in vitamin supplements.

Vitamin A is also found in the drug Accutane, which can help very bad scarring cystic acne and has performed wonders with this condition that were not possible prior to its development.

Q: If someone has a bad reaction to Retin-A and similar products, what else can be used?

A: Alpha hydroxy acids are often used for people who say they can't tolerate Retin-A and its alternatives, because of the way they irritate their skin and make it red. We can use these acids in a stronger concentration than is used for over-the-counter preparations, and we often use it in the office for exfoliation of the skin. We can also combine it with another superficial peel, such as TCA (trichloroacetic acid), and the two together can produce a medium-depth chemical peel.

Q: We have also spoken about topical vitamin C creams that are recommended. Some of these formulas are found in health-food stores or can be purchased on the Internet. Are they the same as the ones you get through your physician?

A: We can't recommend these products because we don't

know what they are or what is in them. Because it is so difficult to stabilize vitamin C in cream form, it is important to use a product that you know will actually deliver the vitamin C to the skin.

Vitamin C creams can help minimize some of the damage done to the skin by years of exposure to sunshine and can also help even out skin tone and improve collagen. These are the main reasons such creams are prescribed for topical use. Also remember that while vitamin C is an antioxidant and is somewhat sun-protective, it should never be used in place of a sunscreen.

Q: What about vitamin E in oils and creams? We have heard for many years that it is useful for healing wounds. Is that true?
A: Vitamin E has positive and negative sides. It is a known sensitizer, meaning that chronic, inconsistent use over a long time could result in an allergic reaction.

In other words, if you use a vitamin E oil or cream for a while, then stop using it, then try it again, or use it one day a week, you can develop a sensitivity or an immune reaction. If this happens, no matter how many years you have used vitamin E products, you may suddenly break out in a very blistery, itchy rash.

Some studies have indicated that vitamin E does not work any better than a moisturizer, so most physicians do not advocate using it. It is an antioxidant, but so is vitamin C, and I recommend that more often.

As for healing scars, there is no scientific proof that vitamin E is any better than a moisturizer. And until we have better studies, we have no reason to think that vitamin E will promote such healing.

Q: You mentioned Kinerase earlier as an emollient for the skin. What does it do?
A: Kinerase is a plant derivative that has been found to reverse some of the damage from sun exposure. It can even out discolored skin tone and can help to fade brown spots caused by the sun. Kinerase can be used as a moisturizer and a photo-rejuvenator that helps minimize some fine lines.

Kinerase does have a beneficial effect, especially when it is used in combination with Retin-A.

Q: How is Kinerase combined with Retin-A?
A: You can use Kinerase in the morning, for example, and Retin-A at night. Retin-A is usually used at night because you don't want to expose Retin-A-treated skin to the sun. You have to use sunblock religiously when using Retin-A because it can degrade when exposed to sunlight.

Retin-A is used to polish up the skin, and makes its surface smoother and more even, so the ultraviolet rays of the sun now have a surface that they can penetrate more easily and intensely.

Q: What about the prescription lightening creams used by dermatologists? Are they effective?
A: Many people develop brown spots on their skin after years of sun exposure. Other people have patches of skin that are darker than others, making the skin look blotchy and unattractive. Sometimes these darker areas are caused by medications such as birth-control pills.

Prescription lightening creams, with the active ingredient hydroquinone, can be very effective in fading these darker spots and creating a more even and smoother skin tone. They usually take a few months to work and patients who are using them have to be very careful to avoid sun exposure.

Occasionally, a physician may prescribe a combination of creams in addition to the hydroquinone, such as cortisone and Retin-A, to help lighten the dark spots. A series of superficial chemical peels can also help make the medicine more effective.

Q: What about the hormone replacement therapy so many women have, which seems to have such rejuvenating effects? Is it also beneficial to the skin?
A: The jury is still out on that one. Especially if someone is not deficient in hormones. Some people think that just as certain amounts of essential fatty acids and cholesterol are needed for healthy skin, hormones are also needed by both men and women. Hormones help to control blood flow and there are hormone receptors throughout the body.

So it is possible that some of the dehydration we see in older people is related to a deficiency of hormones. But we don't have perfect studies saying that this or that specific hormone is beneficial to the skin. And there is also a lot of controversy about possible side effects of hormone replacement therapy, so we will have to wait until we have more scientific information.

Q: What happens when people try to treat their own skin problems and avoid seeing a physician? Can they make things worse?

A: The fact is that the majority of patients with mild acne do not see a physician. And they can do well with over-the-counter treatments and home remedies.

But if the acne starts to get worse and they start to notice scarring or they are becoming very self-conscious and embarrassed about their problem skin and want a quicker fix, they should definitely consult a dermatologist.

Q: What should a person know about self-treating acne?
A: It's best to ask your doctor or pharmacist to recommend an effective product. There are quite a few good products available, including Clearasil and other products with benzoyl peroxide. You have to follow directions very carefully and should wash your hands well after using the product because it is a bleach type of peroxide. If you put it on your hands and don't wash it off and then touch your clothing, you could permanently bleach out the color.

If you use these home acne treatments and see that you are developing more and more craters because your acne is getting deeper, you should really see a doctor. You need to be on pills, medicated creams, or perhaps both.

With serious acne, which is called cystic acne, you develop deep cysts that create deep, permanent scars. One of the best ways to treat this condition is with an oral form of vitamin A medication. But it must be prescribed by a physician who is well versed in treating this condition because of the potential for serious side effects. No woman who is pregnant or of childbearing age can take this medication unless she is also taking birth-control precautions, because it can harm the developing fetus. You also need regular blood tests to make sure your liver and pancreas are not being adversely affected.

Q: What about minor skin problems, such as white-heads on the face? Can you treat those yourself at home?
A: Sometimes people have really tiny whiteheads that no one else even notices, but they bother these people incessantly and they become fixated on them.

Typically, they go to a drugstore and buy some products to get rid of them. They scrub their faces with a buff puff or buy a cleanser with granules in it—such products feel like pumice on the skin—and they keep rubbing and rubbing at the skin, trying to exfoliate and get rid of those whiteheads.

If these people persist, they can develop a condition we call acne mechanica, which means that your actions have created a form of acne. With all your rubbing and abrasion, you have ruptured some of the tiny whiteheads, and by applying pressure, you have created an inflammatory acne out of a noninflammatory acne.

In other words, you used to have little white bumps, but now you have bigger red bumps that can be seen a block away. And once they get inflamed, they can potentially cause scarring.

Q: What happens if you squeeze these bumps?
A: If you squeeze your zits, or "express" them, you may not be doing harm if the contents come out readily, but you are taking a significant risk. Before the contents come out, you could be rupturing the cyst underneath the skin.

This creates deep inflammation that can lead to scarring.

So you have turned a noninflammatory situation into a much more visible and socially embarrassing condition, as well as a potentially scarring situation. It is a big danger and a big concern.

Q: Do people sometimes mistakenly think they have acne?
A: Definitely. Not everything that looks like acne actually is acne. Some conditions that people assume is acne is actually heat rash. Rosacea, a different form of acne, requires different treatment. The apparent acne could also be contact dermatitis, possibly a reaction to a chemical that was on the skin.

It could as well take the form of benign bumps that are composed of enlarged oil glands, which is called sebaceous hyperplasia, or maybe a benign growth of sweat glands, which is called syringoma. There could be benign bumps originating from the epidermis, which is part of a syndrome connected with intestinal polyps.

So you see, you can't always properly diagnose yourself, and it's often wise in these cases to go to a dermatologist so you can be certain about what your skin problems really are. Otherwise, you could treat what you think is acne and make it worse if it's something else. You will also delay getting a proper diagnosis and the treatment you actually need.

Q: Don't some people also borrow medications from their relatives or friends? Can that cause problems?
A: You'd be surprised how often this happens. People

don't want to see a doctor for their skin conditions, so they just use their friends' medications or they use some pills they find in the medicine cabinet at home.

By doing this, they could develop an unwanted side effect that makes the condition worse, such as gram-negative folliculitis (a serious bacterial infection). Then, thinking that their problem is getting worse on its own, they take more pills, which makes it still worse yet.

The paradox is that many times the problem they actually have is very easy to treat, and if they had just gone to a doctor and gotten a proper diagnosis and the correct treatment, it would have cleared up in a few days.

Q: What about using cortisone cream? Can that ever create problems?
A: Yes, if it's used for the wrong condition. Let's say someone has seborrheic dermatitis, which is a scaling, reddish rash that can occur between the nose and the cheek, in the groove along the side of the nose, between the eyebrows, on the eyebrows, on the mustache, beard, around the ears, or on part of the scalp. This condition is socially embarrassing and is sometimes easy to treat and sometimes very difficult to treat.

If someone has seborrhea on their cheeks and they use an over-the-counter cortisone ointment, which is actually a steroid, they run the risk of creating steroid rosacea.

The steroid cream will suppress the inflammation, but at the same time it's creating this type of acne. If they stop using the cortisone cream for a day or two, it naturally gets worse. So if they stop and see it getting worse, they begin to use the cortisone again.

Q: What should people in this situation do?
A: They need to see a dermatologist and they also have to slowly wean themselves off the cortisone. Instead of using it twice a day, use it once a day for a few weeks. Then after that, use it every other day and so on until they can stop using it altogether. In the meantime, they will have received proper medication from the doctor.

In addition, if they do have serious acne, it's good to have it properly diagnosed. A well-trained physician will ask a lot of questions and may uncover other health problems, such as hormonal imbalances or problems with the adrenal or pituitary gland.

Q: What about chronic constipation? Can keeping toxins in your body a long time have a bad effect on your skin?
A: It's very tempting to think that by-products can harm us if they are not excreted properly, but there is no evidence in the medical studies that I'm aware of that indicate a direct correlation between chronic constipation and skin disorders. I don't know if toxins that are in the dried-out stool can leach into the bloodstream and affect the skin. We need more studies to find out if this can occur.

Q: Even though dermatologists can help when there are skin problems, is it possible to have healthy, youthful skin without ever seeing a dermatologist in your lifetime?
A: Yes, absolutely. There are people who live well into their nineties who have done everything a doctor would tell them not to do and who have wonderful skin. A lot

of it is due to inheriting good genes. Some people owe their longevity to a healthy lifestyle, others to their genes, and others to good luck.

Q: What are your final recommendations to people who want to maintain good skin?
A: If you want to take control of your life and increase your statistical chances for maintaining good skin and living a long, healthy life, don't smoke. I can't think of even one serious smoker with good skin.

And of course, protect your skin from the sun. I've had patients who were models and knew from an early age to protect their skin from the sun's rays. There are also people who aren't outdoors a lot, who like to stay inside. Without a doubt, these people have a much less aged appearance.

To Summarize:

- See a board-certified dermatologist if you are concerned about signs of aging skin, unusual spots, discoloration, or have a family history of skin cancer.

- For cosmetic concerns, a dermatologist has a wide range of treatment options.

- Prescription Retin-A and vitamin A products reverse some photo-damage, reduce some lines and wrinkles, increase smoothness, and stimulate collagen growth.

- Alpha hydroxy acids have similar effects, helping exfoliate the skin.

- Vitamin C creams and lotions, which are antioxidants, can minimize sun damage, even out skin tone, and improve collagen.

- Kinerase, a plant derivative, can reverse some sun damage, even out tone, fade brown spots, and moisturize the skin. It can be used in combination with Retin-A.

- Most acne patients do well with over-the-counter products. But self-treating can be risky for more serious acne and other skin disorders.

- Never self-diagnose and use other people's medications. You could cause serious problems, damage your skin, and delay needed treatment.

- You can have healthy, youthful skin for a lifetime without ever seeing a dermatologist if you avoid sun damage, don't smoke, take good care of yourself, and inherit good genes.

Chapter 10

Botox Case Histories

In the following case histories, names and other identifying characteristics have been changed in order to protect the privacy of the patients. In some instances, composites have been created for the purposes of illustration. All medical facts are accurate.

Please remember that all these case histories involve individual, unique cases. No two people are alike and no two people respond in exactly the same way to Botox. These case histories are meant to be informative illustrations and are in no way a guide to the way you may respond to Botox treatment.

Helen: Avoiding a Face-lift

Helen, a thirty-nine-year-old fund-raiser, had her first Botox treatment with another physician about seven months before her first visit to me. She had two rather heavy lines between her eyebrows and three significant horizontal creases on her forehead. Helen made it clear that she did not want to have surgery. She said she was pleased with her previous Botox injections, but felt that the effect was not strong enough and the lines remained too visible.

I gave Helen forty-five units of Botox for the glabellar lines between her eyebrows and also treated the lines across her forehead. When she returned for her next treatment three and a half months later, she told me she was extremely happy with the result, remarking that, "I don't think about a face-lift anymore. I think my face looks great with Botox and it's so much easier and safer than having surgery."

Yvette: A Good but Less-Than-Perfect Result

A thirty-one-year-old social worker, Yvette first came in for Botox after having had fat injections for about three years for the smile creases next to her lips. She was very happy with the results, but was now more aware of the lines between her eyebrows and wanted to do something about them.

Yvette had young-looking skin, but there was a definite line between her brows, even when her face was at rest. She was also concerned that her frequent stress headaches might be related to the way she clenched her face without even realizing it.

Yvette was treated with twenty-five units of Botox in nine different areas on her face, including the bridge of her nose, the corners of her eyebrows, and the areas above the eyebrows. She did not want the numbing cream and told me that she felt only minimal discomfort during the injections.

At her two-week follow-up visit, everything looked

good. Then Yvette returned to the office four and a half months later. We discussed the effect of her first Botox treatment. Although the line between her eyebrows had now markedly diminished, it was still slightly visible and still bothering her.

So for her second treatment, Yvette was given thirty-five units of Botox, a little more than before. When she returned five months later, the effect was still the same, the line was still slightly visible. It is difficult to figure out the reason why additional Botox did not have a better result in making her line disappear completely.

Sometimes we forget how deep a line was originally, in which case, even though the Botox is working, it may not be able to work completely. In some cases, another form of treatment may be required, such as superficial collagen injections. Other people may wait too long between treatments, allowing the muscle to reactivate and create the line again, and then they think they did not get the result they wanted.

Despite the less-than-perfect result, Yvette has been extremely happy with her Botox treatments, telling me, "I love it. Botox is the greatest." In the future, we will try to determine exactly why she is not getting the results she wants and if some other form of treatment can be used in combination with the Botox.

Laura: Weight Loss and Wrinkles

A thirty-year-old librarian, Laura had previously lived in California, where she had undergone microdermabrasion and chemical peels with a dermatologist. She had also tried noninvasive laser treatment to rejuvenate her skin, but saw no visible improvement.

Laura had been overweight and had recently lost about

twenty pounds. She was very happy with the weight loss, but had begun to notice the creases around her eyes, which now seemed more pronounced.

In discussing what she wanted to do, Laura also mentioned that her upper lip seemed too thin and she thought collagen injections might improve it. When Laura confessed that she was a smoker, I encouraged her to try to stop, since the cosmetic effects of smoking are quite negative for the skin and could have been contributing significantly to the lines she now had.

Laura had Botox injections for the crow's-feet lines around her eyes, with nine units on each side in three separate injection areas. But when she returned two weeks later, it was surprising to see that there were hardly any visible results. Explaining that some patients can take up to four weeks or more to achieve the full effect, I advised her to wait a few more weeks.

Laura returned in another two weeks and noted that the lines around her eyes were much better. She realized that the remaining lines were from her big smile muscles, not her eyelid squinting muscles. She then asked to have her forehead treated, and to date, Laura remains very pleased with the effects of Botox.

Audrey: More Units for Thicker Muscles

Audrey had rather deep lines between her brows and was very bothered by them. A fifty-five-year-old graphic designer, she immediately agreed to try Botox treatment and had thirty-five units injected. When she returned a month later, she was very pleased with the results, telling me, "The Botox worked like magic. No more lines!"

Next Audrey wanted to have Botox on her crow's-feet, so we gave her twenty-four units, twelve on each side.

The standard dose is eighteen units, so Audrey was given a larger dose. The reason was that before determining the proper Botox dose for each patient, I ask patients to clench their facial muscles so I can see their lines and compare them against the norm. You can also see their muscles when they do this and judge how thick the muscle is. The thicker the muscle, the more it's been working and the more units that person is going to need.

Audrey's muscles were thicker than average and required a somewhat larger dose of Botox. When she came back for her follow-up visit, we agreed that the results were quite good and the crow's-feet lines were no longer visible.

Martha: Botox Treatment on an Important Day

An outgoing nurse, forty-four-year-old Martha had some fine horizontal creases on her forehead, but in the middle of her brows she had very deep vertical creases, which she strongly disliked.

Martha told me that she had always bruised very easily and was concerned that Botox injections might leave her face black-and-blue. Not knowing that Botox took as long as a few weeks to take full effect, she had come to the office on the same day that she and her husband were going to a special restaurant to celebrate their daughter's high-school graduation.

When I explained the possibility that she might be bruised for this dinner and that she would not have the full results immediately, Martha said she didn't care and wanted the Botox that day. So we injected fifty units of Botox in her forehead and between her eyebrows.

When Martha came back two weeks later, she happily reported, "I didn't have any bruising at all. It was amazing. And the little bumps went away in two hours, so no one knew anything at dinner." In fact, she looked wonderful, but we noticed that she still had a little bit of muscle contraction on the left side of her forehead, so when she comes in at the one-month point for her next treatment, we will add a little Botox to that area to try to make things more symmetrical.

Daniel: A Lifetime Self-improvement Program

A forty-eight-year-old accountant, Daniel was very concerned about his physical appearance and wanted to look his best at all times. He had had liposuction for his "love handles" and worked out a lot, trying to remain in the best possible physical shape.

From childhood, Daniel had always enjoyed outdoor sports, and as a result, he had a lot of sun exposure. He was starting to get worried about the crow's-feet lines around his eyes and asked if Botox would be a good idea.

We talked about the treatment and he decided to go ahead. Daniel required fifteen units of Botox on the crow's-feet lines on each side of his eyes, for a total of thirty units. He experienced no pain or side effects and returned a few weeks later very happy with the results.

Now Daniel is on a regular Botox schedule, coming in about every four or five months as the injections wear off. "I feel about ten years younger since I've tried this stuff," he commented. "And I think my wife is going to be coming in very soon. She never wanted to try Botox before, but I think my appearance has really changed her mind."

Greta: Overcoming Skin Cancer

Following a lifetime of heavy sun exposure, Greta, a fifty-two-year-old physician, developed skin cancer on the side of her nose and had to have it removed. This left her with a rather large hole requiring reconstruction.

An attractive woman, Greta was very concerned about her appearance and anxious to have the area repaired as quickly as possible. She was told that sometimes reconstructive treatments take time to heal completely and that it is important to be patient—the area can even get worse for a while before it starts to get better.

After several follow-up visits and the passage of about a month, the reconstructed area was healing very nicely and Greta felt a lot more confident. She saw that eventually the area would heal and she was now concerned about other areas of her face.

Greta had used Botox in the past, but had experienced some side effects. She had a headache for about a day and later found that her muscles were not even, with more contractile strength and girth on the right side.

So even though she was concerned about the lines on her forehead and wanted to use Botox again, she was also wary of experiencing the same problems.

Two months after her facial reconstruction, Greta came in and the line on her nose was hardly visible, actually healing ahead of schedule. She was extremely pleased and said she now wanted to have Botox on her forehead.

When she was injected, Greta got a smaller amount of Botox on the area with her weaker muscle to try to create an even effect. When she returned two months later, she reported that she'd had no headache after the treatment and felt the results were very even. However, she did notice that her muscle movement was starting to come back, so she had another Botox treatment at that time.

Greta's effects do not seem to last as long as the average person's, but there are no medical concerns involved in treating her with Botox every month or every two months in order to maintain the good effects she wants.

Emily: Improving Every Area

It took Emily, a forty-seven-year-old homemaker, over a year to decide that she wanted cosmetic treatment to improve the deep frown marks between her eyebrows. Once Botox was approved by the FDA for wrinkles, she scheduled a consultation. Since she had been thinking about it for so long, it took her only a minute to decide that she wanted Botox that same day.

Emily had a terrific result and did not bruise or have any side effects, such as headaches. When she came back a few weeks later for her follow-up visit, she remarked, "Everyone says I look so well rested. And I know I look better, so it makes me feel really good about myself."

Emily also said that she had a tendency to frown a lot and now she wasn't able to do it, much to her relief. At her next visit, she decided to treat not only the glabellar area between the brows, but also her crow's-feet and forehead. We used a total of fifty-five units of Botox for these treatments, eighteen on the crow's-feet, twenty-five between the brows, and twelve in the midforehead.

Since she was so pleased with her Botox results, Emily mentioned that she was bothered by her smile folds and asked if Botox could help there. I explained that Botox doesn't work on the smile folds, so we discussed using fat injections, since she thought she might have an allergy to collagen. We will probably proceed with that treatment in the near future.

Betty: Botox Helps Her to Cope

Like Betty, many people have unwanted fine little capillaries or blood vessels around their noses and on their cheeks. A forty-five-year-old hotel manager, Betty initially came to see me to have those capillaries treated, which we did using the V-beam laser. This type of treatment usually requires three to five separate sessions, and while there is definite improvement, it does not always make all the capillaries disappear. Sometimes we need to use a different laser or a different setting, and successful treatment can take time.

After her first laser treatment, Betty asked about Botox. She said she had used it several times in the past with another physician, but after her last treatment had developed a drooping eyebrow on the right side that lasted for four months.

While eyebrows can sometimes droop a little, Betty's effect was pretty extreme in terms of the degree of droop and how long it lasted. This might be explained by a significant underlying difference in the strength of the muscle on the right side. It was also unusual that Betty had had several Botox treatments before with no side effects.

Since she wanted to try Botox again, we did the treatment after talking about possible risks of the same side effect occurring again. Betty had forty units of Botox in her forehead, with fewer on the right side. When she came in three weeks later, she said the Botox had worked for about a week, but the muscle of the right eyebrow was still working a little. Then a week later, everything was fine.

Now Betty has a nice even effect and is very pleased with her appearance. "I may have personal problems sometimes," she told me, "but they stay on the inside. On the outside, I look relaxed, and that helps me to cope better when these problems come up. I'm really happy with the results."

Flora: Close to Complete Success

Flora had no second thoughts about improving her face cosmetically, and by the time she came to see me, she had had collagen for her smile folds as well as Botox with another physician. A thirty-seven-year-old dentist, Flora mentioned that a few days after one previous Botox treatment, she had experienced double vision for a few seconds.

Flora's main concerns were the lines on her forehead and the crow's-feet lines around her eyes. We treated her with forty units of Botox, ten on each side for the crow's-feet and twenty on the lines in her forehead. She also had a fine horizontal crease on her upper lip, so we gave her a total of six units in three different areas there, but the Botox had no effect. A month later we tried a higher dose, twelve units (three units in each of four different areas), again with no result. We could not give her a higher dose because of the risk of affecting her upper-lip function, which can cause drooling.

Flora was very satisfied with the results on her forehead and crow's-feet. She mentioned that she also wanted to get rid of the lines on her upper forehead, and so we treated those.

Flora is continuing with Botox treatment and with collagen for her smile folds. Because she has very dynamic muscles with a lot of movement, she requires more frequent Botox treatments than the average person. "Don't ever let them take this drug away," Flora said. "It does such a fantastic job. Sometimes I can't believe it."

Sebastian: A Face Seen in Public

Because he is in the public eye so much, Sebastian, a fifty-four-year-old politician, is under pressure to look youthful and vibrant. Since his job also involves a lot of pressure, he worried that he allowed the stress to get the better of him and give him frequent stress headaches.

After examining his face, I observed that Sebastian had two deep parallel lines between his eyebrows. In fact, they were so deep that the skin between the grooves actually looked like a protruding bump.

I explained that Botox alone might not be able to give him the kind of smooth effect he was looking for. Years of being stressed and frowning or clenching his face had compounded the problem, and as a result, Sebastian might need collagen injected into the line, plus Botox under-neath. Eventually, he might even need a brow-lift, with a surgeon cutting the muscles to smooth out the lines.

We went ahead with the Botox treatment and gave Sebastian forty-five units of Botox. When he came back in two weeks, the results looked very good and he was extremely pleased. These results lasted about four months, but the line did not go away as much as he wished and it still troubled him.

So when he came for his next treatment, we tried fifty-five units of Botox, a higher dose. This had an even better result and lasted the same amount of time. At that point Sebastian decided that his results were good enough and he was satisfied with his appearance and didn't feel he needed to have any collagen.

Rose: Smiling at the Mirror

Rose came to me because she wanted to look her best for her upcoming wedding. A fifty-three-year-old travel agent, she was marrying for the second "and the last" time and she naturally wanted everything to be perfect.

Rose's main concern was the deep crease between her eyebrows. She said that for many years she had even styled her hair to try to camouflage this area. She said that when she looked in the mirror, all she saw was a huge crease, ruining her face. Now she wanted Botox to get rid of it for her once and for all.

We gave Rose injections of thirty-five units of Botox for her glabellar crease, and within two weeks the lines were almost totally gone. When she returned from her honeymoon and came in for a follow-up visit, she reported that she was now completely happy and actually enjoyed looking in the mirror and not seeing that "hideous groove" anymore.

Fay: Not So Much Like Mother

Sixty-year-old real-estate property manager Fay told me that she had heard about Botox three years ago and had been reading and thinking about it ever since. "I'm very cautious," she said, "and I was concerned about its safety."

Finally convinced of Botox's effectiveness and safety following its FDA approval, Fay came in to improve the deep grooves in her forehead. She mentioned that her mother had the exact same forehead grooves and she wanted to get rid of them.

We gave Fay Botox for her forehead lines, and despite the depth of the grooves, the treatment worked quite well and lasted for about four months. Fay remarked that the injections were much less painful than she had imagined and added that, "The people at work say I look much less stressed and friendlier," noting that the cosmetic effect of Botox treatment seemed to be making her workday a lot more pleasant.

As a result, Fay said she was looking in the mirror more often and was now thinking about what Botox could do for her crow's-feet lines.

Alice: Husband Happy, No More Scowling

After Alice saw a story about Botox on the television news, she wondered if it might be right for her. A sixty-one-year-old dietician, Alice had a deep crease between her eyebrows and had originally thought that silicone might improve it.

However, after Alice did some research on silicone and its possible side effects, she thought Botox was a much better choice and came to us for treatment. Following her Botox injections for the glabellar crease, she was pleased to discover that the treatment was not at all painful and, furthermore, she was no longer able to scowl. "My husband was always complaining about that," she explained.

Like so many satisfied Botox patients, Alice is now considering Botox for another area, the crow's-feet lines around her eyes.

Rhonda: No One Knows What She Did

Convinced that she had a "haggard look," forty-four-year-old Rhonda, a bookkeeper, thought about trying Botox for two years before she finally came to the office. She didn't know exactly what areas needed treatment, so we discussed using Botox on her crow's-feet lines and forehead lines.

Rhonda was eager to make changes in her appearance and went ahead with the Botox treatment immediately, getting a total of forty units in these two locations. She was very pleased with the experience, noting that it didn't hurt or give her a headache, despite her anticipating that it might.

Returning to the office a few weeks later, Rhonda was all smiles. "My friends are all commenting," she said, "and asking me if I changed my hair color or tried some new makeup because they say I look so great. I just smile and don't tell them anything."

In fact, Rhonda's results were quite good and she said that not having the lines on her face anymore made her feel much prettier and more confident about herself.

Joyce: No More Mean Looks

Joyce confided that she always hated her "mean appearance," noting that she didn't feel mean, her face just looked that way. A forty-three-year-old real-estate attorney, she is extremely happy with the results of her Botox treatment.

Joyce was given twenty-five units for the creases between her eyebrows. Fortunately, she is one of those people who have longer-lasting results. After her first Botox injections, she did not need another treatment for five months, and she didn't need her third treatment for six months.

Joyce remarked that now both her clients and colleagues seemed much more relaxed in her presence. "We always got along fine before, but now everything seems so much better. I guess I feel better about myself, too. It's been quite a nice change."

Geraldine: Botox Fever

For the past few years, thirty-two-year-old Geraldine, a public-relations director, had received collagen injections for the glabellar lines between her brows. When she began hearing about Botox, she thought it might be a better choice, so she asked me about it.

Geraldine liked what she heard about Botox and had her first treatment, thirty-five units of Botox for frown lines. She was fine when she left the office, but noticed that she was starting to feel warm as she got home, about half an hour later. She took her temperature and found it was 101. Taking a Tylenol (knowing that Botox patients must avoid aspirin products in the four hours following treatment), Geraldine went to bed earlier than usual, and when she got up the next morning, she felt fine and her temperature was completely normal.

When she reported this to me, I told her that Allergan, the manufacturer of Botox, lists "flulike symptoms" as one of the possible side effects. Of course, there is no way of knowing if her temporary, slight elevation in temperature was caused by Botox or by something else, but it quickly went away.

Other than this minor side effect, Geraldine was thrilled with the results and plans to continue Botox treatments in the future. I also told her that her reaction might have been a onetime occurrence and she might not have it with future Botox treatments.

Carrie: Making Lines in Her Sleep

A retired college professor, sixty-two-year-old Carrie strongly disliked the very deep lines between her brows. She said she thought that when she was asleep, she contracted her face, perhaps contributing to these lines. She suspected this was the case because when she woke up in the morning, she sometimes felt the contraction.

The lines between Carrie's eyebrows were indeed very deep, while the lines around her eyes were not. We treated the glabellar area with forty-five units of Botox, and Carrie was pleased to discover that the effects lasted for about five months. Since then, she has had further Botox and the results have lasted about the same amount of time.

"I'm very happy," she commented. "And when I wake up, I'm no longer clenched. I feel very relaxed and I'm also sleeping better. All thanks to Botox."

Chapter 11

Questions and Answers About Botox

In this chapter, Dr. Shelton answers some questions that people frequently ask about Botox and other cosmetic skin treatments.

Q: I'm twenty-six years old and my skin is pretty good. But I have two older sisters who both have big creases between their brows and lines on their foreheads. I don't want that to happen to me. Could I use Botox to prevent those lines from ever forming?
A: Yes you can, without a doubt. If you were to use Botox on a regular basis, we do think it would prevent those lines from forming. But it is a decision of cost versus merit, and it might be better for you to wait until the lines start forming. There is also a possibility that you will never develop lines like your sisters. However, if you choose to try to prevent them, you could certainly use

Botox on a prophylactic basis if that is what you want to do.

Q: I have a friend whose boyfriend is a medical resident. He has been injecting her with Botox for about a year and she looks great. She told me he would do it for me and I would only have to pay for the Botox. Is there anything wrong with my doing this?
A: It is certainly legal for him to provide you with these Botox shots. Whether or not you should let him inject you is something different. In my opinion, it is always safest and best to have a specially trained and experienced board-certified physician perform your treatment in a medical setting. But the ultimate decision is yours.

Q: I've read all about Botox and understand that it is very safe and has few side effects, but I'm still afraid of it. The idea of a potential poison being injected into my body is frightening. Also the idea of paralyzing muscles—it doesn't seem natural to me. On the other hand, I love the effect and really want to get rid of some of the lines on my face. What should I do?
A: Botox treatment is extremely safe and there has never been a recorded case of anyone developing botulism after using it. Remember that we also use many immunizations, such as those for diphtheria, tetanus, rubella, and measles, and we use them on our children. They are all a very diluted form of potentially toxic diseases, so this method has been around for a long time and has proven to be quite safe. That said, I would not try to coerce you into

doing something you might not want to do, so you really have to come to a decision about this on your own.

Q: I am seventy years old and have heard that Botox has not been tested on people over the age of sixty-five. I am very healthy, see my doctor regularly, don't take any medications, and am very active. I really want to get rid of some of the heavy lines on my face, especially the ones between my brows and on my forehead. Will a doctor give me Botox in spite of my age?
A: Yes. Even though Botox has been thoroughly tested, when the company applied for approval to the FDA, they had to indicate the age range of the people who had been studied. However, these ages do not mean that a physician cannot use the product for people below or above these ages.

But there are some concerns about Botox use with older people. For example, with age there often comes a tendency for the forehead to droop, and if Botox is used in such a case, there could be too much drooping, which could potentially create problems with the eyebrows coming down too low and the eyelids obscuring the field of vision. So you have to see your physician for a consultation and then discuss your individual concerns in order to determine if you are a good Botox candidate.

Q: I have been using collagen for several years to fill in the lines around my mouth and on my forehead. Can I stop using collagen now and switch to Botox?
A: Not entirely. You will have to continue with collagen around the mouth because Botox is not used for those

lines. On your forehead, however, you may be able to completely do away with the use of collagen and substitute Botox injections. You will need to discuss this possibility with your doctor.

Q: Three of my close friends got their first Botox shots at a Botox party. Now they have these parties every few months at their homes. They invited me to the next one, but I don't want to feel pressured to do something when I'm not sure about it. I don't know the doctor they use, either. Do you think I should go to the party?
A: It is always best first to make sure that the doctor is board-certified. You can always choose to go to any meeting, provided you use your common sense, pay attention to your thoughts, and refuse to allow anyone to pressure you into doing something you do not want to do. In addition, we always encourage patients to have their treatments in a clean medical environment, where a physician remains present for supervision following the injections.

Q: I have a very stressful job in television, which I love. I know that I often get upset and angry and also frown quite a bit. Sometimes people even ask me why I'm so upset all the time. Am I creating wrinkles on my face, and if so, what can I do about it?
A: Yes, you are creating wrinkles with your frequent angry or frowning expressions. You might want to make a conscious effort to control these unwanted expressions. And if as a result of making these expressions over the

years you have lines on your face that are troubling you, Botox would probably be the best treatment.

Q: If you use Botox from the time you are in your twenties, will your facial skin stay young looking and never age?
A: No. Botox will not prevent sun damage and the aging effects of prolonged sun exposure. Nor does it prevent lines around the cheeks—those crosshatches that make us look older. But if you protect your face from sun damage and you also use Botox around the eyes and on the forehead, you can certainly minimize the lines that will be created by muscle movement in those areas.

Q: I like my face, lines and all. But my husband says I look much older than him—we are the same age— and he wants me to try Botox. I don't want to lose my husband and don't think I will, but I'm starting to get worried because he keeps nagging me to do it. What should I do?
A: Any elective cosmetic treatment should be done only when people want the treatment themselves. If you are undergoing treatment in order to please someone else, there could be unwanted consequences. For example, if you don't like the results or if you have any side effects, you could be very unhappy with the person who pressured you to have the treatment and you may start to resent and blame that person.

You should also realize that someone who loves you should not coerce you in this way or value you less because of a few lines on your face. It is very important to only undergo cosmetic treatment that *you* want, not that someone else wants.

Q: I'm a thirty-five-year-old woman and my skin is very smooth and tight. I'm afraid that if I lose the forty pounds that my doctor told me to lose, my skin will get loose and saggy. What is your opinion about this?
A: If your doctor is telling you to lose forty pounds, there are obvious cardiac risks in your being overweight. These risks far outweigh any cosmetic concerns, because the reality is that it doesn't matter how good you look if you're in a coffin.

So I advise you to lose the weight and then deal with any consequences afterward. For some people, there is a sagging effect after a big weight loss, but there are procedures that can greatly improve it, whether it's minimally invasive fat injections or a surgical neck-lift or face-lift.

Q: Every two weeks I have my hair done at a local beauty salon. Recently, one of the makeup people started giving Botox shots. When the women who had treatments came back in two weeks, they all looked great. The cost is reasonable, so I'm thinking of doing it. Is it legal?
A: I don't know. You will have to check your local laws to find out if it is legal for nonmedical personnel to administer Botox at your beauty salon. But it is definitely unwise and potentially dangerous.

Only trained medical professionals should give Botox

treatments. Botox is not makeup. It is a prescription drug that must be used carefully by a physician. Aside from the legal and ethical considerations, Botox administered by someone without proper medical credentials could result in unwanted side effects, like a persistent droopy eye or long-lasting headaches. If you want to use Botox, see your doctor.

Q: I'm a forty-three-year-old man in a very high-profile position. I have to appear in public quite often and many people are familiar with my looks. In the past, I've often told people that I'm completely against plastic surgery and I still feel the same way, but my skin is now beginning to show signs of aging. If I use Botox, will people immediately know that I did something or can the changes be made to look more subtle?
A: Without a doubt, the effects of Botox can be adjusted based on your desires and the physician's talents. You do not need to end up with a "mask" for a face just because you use Botox. There can be select targeting of individual muscle groups and your appearance can still look quite natural.

Q: My face is lopsided, with one eyebrow higher than the other and the corner of my mouth on the right side drooping lower than the corner on the left. These things are really very slight, but they have bothered me for a long time. Could Botox correct them and even things out?
A: Yes, Botox can help to create a more even effect on your face. But we have to know the reason why your face

is uneven. Some people have neurologic conditions that have affected their nerve-muscle interplay and there can be significant differences between the two sides of their faces. Using Botox to create a symmetric or equal look requires technical skill, but many doctors will be able to do this. As for your mouth, you might consider seeing a neurologist who is adept at using Botox to see if a more equal look can be achieved.

Q: I'm nineteen and have marks on my face from acne. Can Botox get rid of them?
A: Probably not.

Most acne scars of recent origin can be improved with nondestructive (nonablative) lasers, which help remove the color or redness, making them less apparent. These are the shallow scars, the ones that respond best to this type of laser.

Ablative lasers, which are more aggressive, can give an even better effect, especially with older scars, but these also present some risks of permanent scarring. Another option is to have pitted scars surgically removed and replaced with small samples of skin, called punch grafts, which are applied prior to laser resurfacing. You really have to consult with your doctor to find out which treatment is best for your particular acne scars.

Q: I'm a fifty-seven-year-old grandfather and recent widower. After a year of mourning, I want to start living again and would like to have some of my wrinkles removed so I will feel better about myself before I start dating. My children are very upset about this

and tell me I will ruin my character and won't be the same person anymore. What do you think?

A: People have to live with themselves, and ultimately they need to do what they think is right while utilizing advice from family members and friends. They should listen to what others have to say, think about it in earnest, and then make their own decisions.

No one should rush in and have an elective procedure without thinking about it first. You should look into the facts and become familiar with the risks, because every procedure has risks. You always have to weigh the risks and the benefits and see which side is stronger for you.

When you make your own decision after educating yourself, your family needs to be supportive. So if you decide to have Botox treatment, your family should support your decision. Even if there is a side effect or complication or you or they are not happy with the results, the family needs to stick by you, because that's the role of a family. You might also want to remind them that the effects of Botox wear off in a few months, so if you decide to use it, they should probably reserve judgment for a while.

Q: **If vitamin C is good for your skin in creams and lotions, why isn't it also good as a vitamin supplement? Isn't the excess just excreted and isn't it good to bathe the cells in an antioxidant to fight the effects of aging?**

A: It is true that vitamin C helps to nourish the skin and fortify blood vessels. However, it can only do this if it is integrated into the epidermis, an effect that is not seen as much when vitamin C is taken internally rather than applied externally. In addition, the photo-protective proper-

ties of the vitamin are best obtained by using topical
preparations that are applied directly onto the skin. Finally, while it is true that unneeded vitamin C is excreted,
there is also some evidence that vitamin C can contribute
to kidney stones if taken in excess.

**Q: I tried Botox once and loved it, but I also got a
droopy eyelid that lasted for a few weeks. Now I'm
afraid to try it again. My friend went to a different
doctor and got great results. Should I try that doctor
instead?**
A: Just because you got a lowered eyelid once, it doesn't
necessarily mean that you will get the same effect if you
use Botox again. The statistical risk of an eyelid lowering
is between 2 and 5 percent or more.

If the Botox used by one physician is diluted more than
the Botox used by another physician, the physician who
dilutes more must give you a greater amount of solution
to equal the same number of units. That greater volume
of solution may diffuse behind the muscle, due to gravity,
and affect the eyelid muscle that keeps the eyelid up.

The problem could also be technique. If the lowest percent of an eyelid lowering is 2 percent, that means the
busiest physicians administering the most Botox may, in
fact, have a higher absolute number of complications than
someone else who is doing less Botox. That's because the
busier physician is seeing more patients.

All of this means that you don't necessarily need to see
a different physician. In fact, a new physician would be
somewhat handicapped, not knowing exactly what was
done previously. You should begin by going back to the
doctor who gave you Botox, discuss the side effect, and

try to find the cause. There may be a good reason for it that can be avoided in future treatments, but you can only find out by returning to that first physician.

Q: I have a deep cleft in my chin that I hate. Can Botox take it away? If not, what can?
A: Botox can minimize the cleft, but it will probably not make it go away altogether. An augmentation could be done underneath your skin with different substances, such as fat injections or even a permanent implant. You should see a qualified physician for a consultation to discuss the recommended options.

Q: Would someone who has had a face-lift ever have a reason to use Botox?
A: A face-lift typically does not address the forehead. If someone has had a brow-lift and a face-lift, there may be less need for Botox in the forehead. There may be even less need for Botox between the eyebrows if you have had an extensive brow-lift.

However, even those patients who have undergone this type of surgery may, in fact, have a partial recurrence of those creases. In this event, Botox can be of help. In addition, a face-lift and brow-lift do not typically treat the lines around the eyelids, and for that reason, crow's-feet lines could still benefit from Botox treatment.

Q: I had a moderate case of botulism from food poisoning several years ago. I'm fine now, but wonder if it is safe for me to use Botox.

A: If you have had botulism in the past it does not increase the risk for side effects from Botox injections. However, there is a possibility that the botulism may have caused your body to create antibodies. If that is the case, Botox may not work well.

Q: I've heard that you can get shots of Botox under your arms before an important social event and you will not perspire. Is that true, and if so, is it safe?
A: Botox is safe, and yes, it is true. However, it does not mean that one treatment is enough. There are times when patients will need to come back for a second treatment after the area is rechecked for persistent islands of sweat glands that are still functioning. So keep in mind that because it may take several days for the Botox to be effective and because you may need a second treatment, you should not have Botox for heavy perspiration just a day or two before your social event.

Furthermore, the number of units needed for this type of treatment tends to be quite high as compared with the number used in cosmetic treatments for facial lines. And since most insurance companies do not cover this treatment, you should be sure to discuss the cost prior to agreeing to have the procedure done.

Q: I had a Botox treatment and then found out I was pregnant. My doctor said there probably won't be any bad effects on my baby, but I'm still worried. Is there anything I should do?
A: You should discuss your concerns with your obstetrician and perhaps with a pediatrician as well. But there

have been no cases of pediatric malformation attributed to Botox that was inadvertently given to pregnant women.

Even so, it is very important to remember that no one who is pregnant should willingly have Botox treatment. Nor should any physician administer Botox to a woman who is known to be pregnant, since scientific studies have not been done to prove that there is absolutely no danger.

Q: Botox has only been used cosmetically for a little more than a decade, so I wonder if there is any chance that after twenty or thirty years or more, we could discover that it has unwanted long-term side effects.
A: Remember that Botox has been used for more than twenty years for neuromuscular and ophthalmologic conditions—in larger doses than we use cosmetically—and we have not seen any long-term conditions or side effects. Of course, there is always a chance that we may learn of some unexpected long-term side effects in the future, but at this point Botox appears very safe.

Q: Can using Botox increase my self-esteem? I sometimes worry a lot about my appearance and think that people don't find me attractive. I have some wrinkles around my eyes that make me look older, especially when I laugh or smile. They really don't bother me too much, but I worry about what other people think. Should I try Botox to get rid of them?
A: If the lines that are bothering you are significant enough to be noticed by other people, and you think that they are viewing these lines in a negative way, it may be

worthwhile for you to at least try Botox, since it is a safe treatment.

Botox can definitely increase your self-confidence, making you feel more socially at ease and cheerful. Some Botox patients report that they are far more outgoing in the presence of others and that people now find them more enjoyable to be around. The decision is yours, of course, but yes, Botox can increase self-esteem for many people.

Q: I have heard that some people who used Botox died afterward. Is that true?
A: Allergan, the manufacturer of Botox, is aware of a few rare deaths in patients who have had Botox treatments sometime before their demise. In some cases, these patients had significant health problems that may have caused their deaths. So far, no deaths have been attributed to the use of Botox itself.

Q: If people frown a lot and get lines in their faces, shouldn't they see a therapist instead of a dermatologist? If they use Botox, won't the personal problems that made them frown still remain untreated?
A: If their frowning is related solely to some personal problem, then seeking professional help might be a good idea. However, even though the lines between the eyebrows are called "frown lines," they are not necessarily caused by frowning, stress, or being upset. They can also result from being puzzled or inquisitive or even chronically happy!

Q: I'm a forty-two-year-old businesswoman and I tried Botox a month ago, just for fun. I was curious to see what would happen. Now I've gotten so many compliments from people—most of whom don't even know what I did—that I'm afraid I will become addicted to Botox and will need to keep using it to remain looking as good as I do now. Is there such a thing as Botox addiction and could it be a problem?

A: I have never seen this to be a problem with any of my patients. If someone stops using Botox, the lines do not come back worse than they were before. There is a gradual transition, because the lines start to improve if someone has used Botox regularly for a while. And if people like the effects of Botox, then they can continue the treatments. I am not aware of any physical addiction that has ever developed.

You may certainly desire to continue your Botox treatments indefinitely. It is quite possible that you will have a difficult time emotionally if you stop the treatments for such reasons as financial concerns and see your wrinkles return. But I have not heard of any people with psychological addictions to Botox.

Q: I have heard that Botox treatment only takes a few minutes, so I'm thinking of having it during my lunch hour. Is it really true that I can have Botox and then go right back to work?

A: Provided you are not physically active at work and that you do not have to bend over in the four hours after treatment, then you can return to work. However, the Botox treatment may leave temporary small red swellings at the injection sites that will go down over a period of an hour or sometimes more.

Some patients do not have any bumps, but if it is important for you to go back to work, you should be aware that you may have them on your face. No one can guarantee what immediate results you will have following your Botox treatment, so it may be best for you to schedule your appointment at the end of your workday.

Q: Isn't all this cosmetic treatment with Botox and other drugs just vanity? Isn't it more important to do the most you can with your life and grow old gracefully, wrinkles and all? By advocating things like Botox, aren't we telling ourselves and our children that physical appearance and looking young at all costs is the most important thing in life?

A: That is an excellent question and one that deserves serious consideration. First of all, we are all very fortunate to live in a free and technologically advanced society where many luxuries, including cosmetic treatments, are available to us. People are individuals and deserve the freedom of choice to use these treatments and improve their physical appearance if they wish to.

For some people, looking better makes them feel better—it improves their outlook on life. Feeling better about themselves can influence everything else in their lives, such as how they relate to others, how they perform at work, and even, simply, how they live their lives.

When we look at people, the first place we look is the face. It is expressive and how it looks can make us feel friendly or cautious or fearful toward another person. Just as a beautiful painting can attract us and elevate our spirit, so can a beautiful face.

But it's also true that faces with lines and wrinkles can be just as or even more beautiful than smooth, ageless faces, depending on who is viewing that face and how he or she feels about the person and the aesthetics.

So there are many factors involved in deciding to take advantage of cosmetic treatments. These treatments are available and we must allow people to make their own decisions and then respect those decisions.

When it comes to sun damage, you have to remember that many years ago, people were not aware of the harmful effects of sun's rays on the skin. As a result, large numbers of people overexposed their skin and are now faced with unwanted wrinkles and skin cancers. I don't think it is vanity to use modern technology to try to reverse some of the damage and signs of aging that people created without realizing what they were doing.

Finally, as a dermatologist, I enjoy working with my hands and trying to improve people's skin. About half of my practice is devoted to skin cancer, and I get a lot of satisfaction from performing reconstructive surgery. I love it when I see how often a beautiful result can occur with an almost imperceptible scar.

When some of my skin-cancer patients see these results, they suddenly realize that cosmetic treatments can be quite wonderful. That's when they begin asking about Botox and collagen and other treatments. Because almost everyone wants to look more youthful.

If you could see how happy people are when they see their skin-cancer scars fade or that the big bulge between their eyebrows or the turkey-gobbler neck that they have hated for years is suddenly gone, you would not call it vanity.

Just by using these techniques, you can change people's perceptions of themselves almost overnight. They have a new level of self-confidence, they are happier and friendlier, more sociable, and sometimes have better relationships. Your physical appearance is profoundly connected to your personality, and when you like what you see in the mirror, it can dramatically improve your life.

No one should ever be coerced into having a cosmetic treatment. But if they do want it and the results are positive, I don't see why anyone else should object. If you could see how people's spirits are lifted, you would realize that cosmetic treatments are not just vain and empty procedures. They have many, many worthwhile merits.

Q: What is your final word on Botox?
A: Botox is a safe, quick, and effective treatment that can take years off your face. It is noninvasive, has very few side effects, and is a giant leap over similar cosmetic treatments of the past. I encourage anyone who is interested to investigate Botox further with a qualified physician, and if they want, to try it. If you don't like your results, they will quickly wear off. If you do like your results, you may well find Botox to be a major asset to your life.

Conclusion

Since April 2002, when the FDA approved Botox treatment for glabellar lines or the creases between the eyebrows, followed by an expensive advertising campaign launched by its manufacturer, Allergan, the use of this drug has soared.

In the year 2000, Botox treatments represented 20 percent of all cosmetic procedures performed by surgeons in this country. With an estimated 1.6 million Americans using Botox by 2001—up 45 percent in just one year—some experts are now predicting that by 2006, as many as a billion people may be using it.

With virtually unprecedented popularity and appeal to so many people, Botox may now be considered one of a select group of "blockbuster" drugs, in a class with Viagra, Prilosec, and Vioxx in terms of its widespread use.

But Botox, unlike these other drugs, is not meant to treat people with a specific health disorder. Its appeal is much broader than that, and as word of its effectiveness spreads, it's likely that more and more people will want to try it—at least once.

At the moment Botox is especially popular with women between the ages of thirty-five and fifty. This group represented more than half of all cosmetic Botox patients in 2001. But the number of men, who now represent around 15 percent of Botox patients, appears to be increasing, as is the number of people under the age of thirty-five (also currently about 15 percent). And celebrities, who used Botox quietly in the past, are now beginning to speak out and acknowledge that this drug is the reason why they look so great.

The message? Today, no one has to have old-looking skin. By having just a few Botox shots every three or four months, you can put off having a brow-lift for years—maybe forever. With ten or twenty minutes in the doctor's office, and minimal side effects that quickly wear off, you can instantly take five or more years off your face. Chances are, no one will even realize what you did, unless you choose to tell them.

You will look more relaxed, refreshed, self-confident, and happy. People will find you more approachable, and as an added bonus, you may also find that your tension headaches have disappeared.

It's true that some people look down on Botox and other cosmetic skin treatments as nothing more than signs of vanity, but why should there be anything wrong with trying to look your best?

If you go to a party or special event, no one will criticize you for dressing nicely or putting on some special jewelry or makeup. If you have your nails done, try a new hairstyle at the beauty parlor, or buy the latest night cream at a department store, you will not come under attack from your friends. So why should using Botox be so different?

For many people, Botox is indeed a miracle that has changed their lives. After all, your face is the first thing most people see, and it is an important influence on the way we interact, relate to one another, and make judgments about one another.

Ask yourself: Do you know anyone who would rather see an angry, frowning, sun-damaged face than a pleasant, relaxed, vibrant face?

Botox allows us to look younger without spending a lot of time, money, or downtime. With no invasive or risky surgery, we can now take years off our faces—and our psyches—just by spending a few minutes every few months in the doctor's office.

It's true: Botox may not be for everyone. As we've seen, it can't improve many types of skin problems.

Of course, there are many people who don't want any part of Botox. They're happy with their faces, lines and all—even proud of them as "signs of character," or marks of the long life they've lived. And there's certainly nothing wrong with that.

But for the rest of us, Botox can really be a wonder.

So perhaps someday you will be one of those people looking in the mirror and saying, "I love this stuff, I absolutely love it."

Resources

The following organizations will help you find a qualified Botox doctor in your area. They will also provide further information about Botox and other cosmetic skin treatments.

The American Society for Dermatologic Surgery
5550 Meadowbrook Drive, Suite 120
Rolling Meadows, IL 60008
Phone: 847-956-0900
Web site: *www.aboutskinsurgery.com*

The American Academy of Dermatology
930 East Woodfield Road
Schaumberg, IL 60173
Phone: 847-330-0230
Web site: *www.skincarephysician.com/agingskinnet*

American Academy of Cosmetic Surgery
737 North Michigan Avenue, Suite 820
Chicago, IL 60611
Phone: 312-981-6760
Web site: *www.cosmeticsurgery.org*

American Society of Plastic Surgeons and Plastic
Surgery Education Foundation
444 East Algonquin Road
Arlington Heights, IL 60005
Phone: 847-228-9900
Web site: *www.plasticsurgery.org*

Allergan Inc. (manufacturer of Botox)
P.O. Box 19534
2525 Dupont Drive
Irvine, CA 92612
Phone: 800-347-4500; 714-246-4500
Fax: 714-246-6987
Web site: *www.botox.com*